STANDARDS FOR HEALTH SERVICES IN JUVENILE DETENTION AND CONFINEMENT FACILITIES

2011

These standards represent the official position of the National Commission on Correctional Health Care with respect to requirements for health services in juvenile detention and confinement facilities. They do not necessarily represent the official position of supporting organizations or individuals represented on the National Commission on Correctional Health Care Board of Directors.

National Commission on Correctional Health Care
1145 W. Diversey Parkway, Chicago, IL 60614
www.ncchc.org

ISBN 0-929561-24-4

TABLE OF CONTENTS

ACKNOWLEDGMENTS

Many individuals have contributed to this edition of *Standards for Health Services in Juvenile Detention and Confinement Facilities*. The National Commission on Correctional Health Care appreciates the efforts of all who have been involved. Much credit must be given to NCCHC's Juvenile Health Committee, which spearheaded the revision effort. The committee began its work in the latter part of 2009, soliciting and receiving a large number of suggestions and comments from correctional health professionals, facility administrators, and national associations in the health, corrections, and legal fields. The committee carefully reviewed every response and, over the course of meetings, independent research, and follow-up correspondence, crafted these standards.

During the revision process, members of the Juvenile Health Committee were as follows:

Judith P. Robbins, LCSW, JD, CCHP-A, Chair; liaison, National Association of Social Workers; Director, Juvenile Detention Mental Health Program, Yale Behavioral Health/Yale Medical School, Department of Psychiatry, New Haven, Connecticut

Patricia N. Reams, MD, MPH, CCHP, Vice-Chair; liaison, American Academy of Pediatrics; Pediatrician, Access Now, Richmond Academy of Medicine, Richmond, Virginia

Vickie Alston, LCSW, QICW; Health Services Administrator/Manager of Transitional Services, University of Connecticut Health Center, Correctional Managed Health Care, Farmington, Connecticut

Paula Braverman, MD; Cincinnati Children's Hospital Medical Center, Division of Adolescent Medicine, Cincinnati, Ohio

Catherine A. Gallagher, PhD; Professor, George Mason University, Department of Public and International Affairs, Fairfax, Virginia

Lindsay M. Hayes, MS; Project Director, National Center on Institutions and Alternatives, Mansfield, Massachusetts

Steven J. Helfand, PsyD, CCHP; Regional Vice President, Correct Care Solutions, Nashville, Tennessee

Charlotte Kent, PhD, MPH; Chief, Epidemiology Unit, Centers for Disease Control and Prevention, Atlanta, Georgia

Robert E. Morris, MD, CCHP; liaison, Society for Adolescent Health and Medicine; Professor of Pediatrics, Department of Pediatrics, University of California, Los Angeles, California

Joseph V. Penn, MD, CCHP; liaison, American Academy of Child and Adolescent Psychiatry; Director, Mental Health Services, University of Texas Medical Branch Correctional Managed Care, Huntsville, Texas

Ronald E. Persing, MD; Assistant Professor, University of Mississippi Medical Center, Jackson, Mississippi

Ellyn R. Presley, RN, CCHP-RN; Health Services Administrator, Prince William County Juvenile Detention Center, Manassas, Virginia

David W. Roush, PhD; liaison, National Juvenile Detention Association; Director, Juvenile Justice Associates, LLC, Albion, Michigan

Michelle Staples-Horne, MD, MPH, CCHP; Medical Director, Georgia Department of Juvenile Justice, Decatur, Georgia

Ohiana Torrealday, PhD, CCHP; Administrative Director, University of Texas Medical Branch, Austin, Texas

Ana M. Viamonte Ros, MD, MPH; liaison, Association of State and Territorial Health Officials; Florida Surgeon General and Secretary, Department of Health, Tallahassee, Florida

Patricia Voermans, MSN, APNP, CCHP-RN; liaison, American Nurses Association; Health Services Consultant, Wisconsin Department of Corrections, Madison, Wisconsin

Barbara A. Wakeen, MA, LD, CCHP; liaison, American Dietetic Association; Dietitian, Correctional Nutrition Consultants, North Canton, Ohio

Ronald Wiborg, MA, MBA; liaison, National Association of Counties, Senior Program Manager, Hennepin County Department of Human Services and Public Health, Minneapolis, Minnesota

The revision of the juvenile standards also benefitted from the special efforts of a number of individuals. B. Jaye Anno, PhD, CCHP-A, senior partner, Consultants in Correctional Care, Santa Fe, New Mexico, added her considerable expertise to the process. Other experts who helped include Carl C. Bell, MD, CCHP, liaison, National Medical Association, Director, Institute for Juvenile Research, Chicago, Illinois; Nina Dozoretz, MA, RHIA, CCHP, Immigration Health Services, Washington, DC; Thomas J. Fagan, PhD, liaison, American Psychological Association, Nova Southeastern University, Fort Lauderdale, Florida; Kevin Fiscella, MD, MPH, liaison, American Society of Addiction Medicine, University of Rochester School of Medicine and Dentistry, Rochester, New York; and Robert L. Hilton, RPh, CCHP, liaison, American Pharmacists Association, Aurora, Missouri. Wayne Liddell, MS, Berrien Center, Michigan, and Ronald M. Shansky, MD, MPH, Chicago, Illinois, lent their expertise to the development of the performance measures. In addition, the following professionals lent help through comments and suggestions during the early phase of revision: Judith F. Cox, MA, CCHP, Clifton Park, New York, and Patrick A. Sheridan, MD, MBA, CCHP, Frankfort, Kentucky.

NCCHC's Policy and Standards Committee reviewed and approved the final draft of the *Standards* and presented it to the Board of Directors for adoption. Committee members included Renee Kanan, MD, Chair, liaison, American College of Physicians; Peter C. Ober, PA-C, JD, CCHP, Vice-Chair, liaison, American Academy of Physician Assistants; Carl C. Bell, MD,

CCHP, liaison, National Medical Association; Robert Cohen, MD, liaison, American Public Health Association; Eileen F. Couture, DO, CCHP, liaison, American College of Emergency Physicians; Joseph E. Paris, MD, CCHP-A, liaison, Society of Correctional Physicians; Peter Perroncello, CJM, CCHP, liaison, American Jail Association; Alvin J. Thompson, MD, liaison, American Medical Association; and Henry C. Weinstein, MD, CCHP, liaison, American Psychiatric Association.

The revision was coordinated by NCCHC staff: R. Scott Chavez, PhD, MPA, CCHP-A, Vice President; Matissa Sammons, Juvenile Health Committee liaison; and Jennifer E. Snow, MPH, CCHP, Director of Accreditation. Editing was completed by Jaime Shimkus, Editor, and Paula J. Hancock, MEd, CCHP, Director of Professional Services.

Many others also contributed to this publication through a call for public comments. We are grateful for the efforts of everyone who participated, since the result promises to promote improved health services in our nation's juvenile detention and confinement facilities.

Edward A. Harrison, CCHP
President
National Commission on Correctional Health Care
April 2011

MEMBERS OF THE 2011 NCCHC BOARD OF DIRECTORS

David W. Roush, PhD
National Juvenile Detention Association

Jayne Russell, MEd, CCHP-A
Academy of Correctional Health
Professionals

Ryung Suh, MD
American College of Preventive Medicine

Alvin J. Thompson, MD
American Medical Association

Ana Viamonte Ros, MD
Association of State and Territorial Health
Officials

Patricia Voermans, MSN, CCHP-RN
American Nurses Association

Barbara A. Wakeen, RD, CCHP
American Dietetic Association

Henry C. Weinstein, MD, CCHP
American Psychiatric Association

Nancy B. White, LPC
American Counseling Association

Ronald Wiborg, MBA
National Association of Counties

HOW TO USE THIS BOOK

These standards represent NCCHC's requirements for health services in juvenile detention and confinement settings. They are intended for use in evaluating the health services in facilities of all sizes, including those that are part of larger systems. Juvenile correctional systems may find the standards helpful in directing their operations. State governments contracting with community or private agencies for health services may find the standards useful for specifying contract expectations and evaluating contract performance. Once implemented, the standards can lead to increased efficiency of health services delivery, greater organizational effectiveness, better overall health protection for juveniles, reduced risk of liability related to health services, and NCCHC health services accreditation.

This manual contains 70 standards grouped under 9 general areas: Section A – Governance and Administration (12 standards), Section B – Safety (6 standards), Section C – Personnel and Training (9 standards), Section D – Health Care Services and Support (5 standards), Section E – Juvenile Care and Treatment (13 standards), Section F – Health Promotion (5 standards), Section G – Special Needs and Services (11 standards), Section H – Health Records (4 standards), and Section I – Medical-Legal Issues (5 standards).

Every standard is categorized, numbered, and named. For example, in Y-A-01 Access to Care, the "Y" designation means these standards apply to juvenile facilities (in the jail and prison manuals, the respective designations are "J" and "P"), the second letter ("A") refers to the topical section to which the standard belongs, and the number refers to its position within that section.

The statement below the standard's name is designated as the standard, a succinct sentence or two about the topic and statement of the expected outcome. Following the standard are compliance indicators, which specify how meeting the standard can usually be assessed. Next is the discussion section, the first sentence of which states the intent of the standard. The compliance indicators and statement of intent are the essence of what is required to meet the standard.

The discussion section can serve several purposes. It is sometimes used to further explain the intent of the standard or its compliance indicators. The discussion section may also define terms, give guidance to compliance, refer to other resources, and explain applicability for special circumstances. For words in italics, definitions appear in the discussion or glossary.

Seven standards have performance measures. These are measurable goals the facility may use to assess compliance with the intent of the standards. These measures can assist the CQI program in evaluating quantitative and qualitative outcomes. Achieving the goals of the performance measures is desirable and encouraged, but it is not required for accreditation purposes. See Appendix B – Compliance Indicators and Performance Measures for further guidance.

Finally, a number of standards contain a section labeled "optional recommendations." As the name suggests, following the recommendations is not required in order to be in compliance with the standard but may be beneficial to some systems.

Because the standards are developed for correctional health care systems, some aspects of care are addressed in more than one standard. For instance, standard Y-G-01 Chronic Disease Services provides guidance on the treatment of chronic disease patients, whereas identifying inmates with a disease is an issue addressed in the standards Y-E-02 Receiving Screening, Y-E-04 Health Assessment, and Y-E-07 Nonemergency Health Care Requests Services. Furthermore, many other standards speak to the system that should be in place for chronic disease services to be effective; for example, Y-A-02 Responsible Health Authority, Y-A-03 Medical Autonomy, and Y-E-12 Continuity of Care During Incarceration.

Each standard is classified as either "essential" or "important," designations that represent categories used in NCCHC's accreditation program. For an explanation of these categories, and of the accreditation program in general, see Appendix D – NCCHC Accreditation.

To further assist the reader, an appendix includes additional information and resources for certain topics, including an explanation of NCCHC's accreditation process.

CHANGES MADE SINCE THE STANDARDS WERE LAST PUBLISHED

The 2011 edition of the *Standards* features several changes from the previous edition.

Two new standards were added:
- Y-B-03 Patient Safety
- Y-B-04 Staff Safety

In four instances, two or more standards were combined:
- Standard Y-B-01 Infection Control Program contains elements previously found in Ectoparasite Control (formerly Y-B-04).
- Standard Y-B-02 Environmental Health and Safety contains elements previously found in Kitchen Sanitation and Food Handlers (formerly Y-B-03).
- Standard Y-H-04 Management of Health Records contains elements previously found in Availability and Use of Health Records (formerly Y-H-04), Transfer of Health Records (formerly Y-H-05), and Retention of Health Records (formerly Y-H-06).
- Standard Y-I-04 Informed Consent and Right to Refuse contains elements previously found in Informed Consent (formerly Y-I-04) and Right to Refuse Treatment (formerly Y-I-05).

Some changes to the standards were substantive, while others were more subtle. Standards that were extensively revised include the following:
- Y-A-03 Medical Autonomy
- Y-A-04 Administrative Meetings and Reports
- Y-A-05 Policies and Procedures
- Y-A-06 Continuous Quality Improvement Program
- Y-A-09 Privacy of Care
- Y-A-10 Procedure in the Event of a Juvenile Death
- Y-B-02 Environmental Health and Safety
- Y-C-01 Credentialing
- Y-C-02 Clinical Performance Enhancement
- Y-C-04 Health Training for Child Care Workers
- Y-C-09 Orientation for Health Staff
- Y-D-01 Pharmaceutical Operations
- Y-D-02 Medication Services
- Y-D-03 Clinic Space, Equipment, and Supplies
- Y-E-02 Receiving Screening
- Y-E-04 Health Assessment
- Y-E-12 Continuity of Care During Incarceration
- Y-G-01 Chronic Disease Services
- Y-G-05 Suicide Prevention Program
- Y-I-01 Restraint and Seclusion

There was one change in status:
- Important to Essential: Y-G-01 Chronic Disease Services

Finally, the order of the standards has been changed slightly; for example, Y-B-06 Procedure in the Event of Sexual Assault was formerly Y-G-09.

GUIDELINES FOR DISEASE MANAGEMENT

A guideline for disease management is a consensus statement designed to help practitioners and their patients make decisions about appropriate health care for specific clinical circumstances. The guidelines contain information and evidence-based recommendations on the best practices for the clinical management of specific health conditions.

NCCHC's guidelines are important because they aim to standardize, guide, and improve clinical practice in correctional institutions. They are based on nationally accepted science and practice, and take into consideration special circumstances commonly found in correctional facilities. The guidelines are reviewed annually and, if necessary, updated to reflect the latest evidence-based practices. Guidelines have been developed for conditions common among incarcerated adults and juveniles.

The guidelines can be accessed online at www.ncchc.org.

POSITION STATEMENTS

In addition to promulgating standards, NCCHC periodically adopts position statements on topics of importance for the correctional health care field. The position statements are of interest to correctional administrators and health professionals because they offer recommendations on a wide range of health-related issues. They can be of interest to policy makers and the public because they often frame the social, economic, and political aspects of contemporary correctional health care issues. NCCHC's position statements can be accessed online at www.ncchc.org.

JUVENILE FACILITIES SEEKING ACCREDITATION

Juvenile detention and confinement facilities that follow the standards should seek to be accredited. NCCHC accreditation provides an independent, professional assessment of compliance with the standards and has proven to be an effective tool in achieving and maintaining peak organizational performance.

The compliance indicators listed in each standard are the same measures used by accreditation surveyors when they come on site. Compliance may be verified through health record reviews, observation, interviews, and other information-gathering methods. On-site reviews are often quite collegial, and our expert accreditation survey team members may offer suggestions for improvement based on their many years of correctional health care experience.

NCCHC is not a membership organization and there are no requirements to becoming accredited other than meeting the standards and adhering to NCCHC accreditation policies. Juvenile facilities of all sizes have been accredited using NCCHC standards. The smallest have fewer than 20 residents. Many standards take into account the size of the juvenile population.

For a more in-depth discussion of the accreditation process, please see Appendix D. For clarification of any of the standards or their applicability to your facility, an evaluation of compliance, or other technical assistance, please contact us.

National Commission on Correctional Health Care
1145 W. Diversey Parkway
Chicago, Illinois 60614
Phone: 773-880-1460
Fax: 773-880-2424
Email: accreditation@ncchc.org
www.ncchc.org

SECTION A – GOVERNANCE AND ADMINISTRATION

Y-A-01
essential

ACCESS TO CARE

Standard

Juveniles have *access to care* to meet their serious medical, dental, and mental health needs.

Compliance Indicator

The responsible health authority (RHA) identifies and eliminates any barriers to juveniles receiving health care.

Definition

Access to care means that, in a timely manner, a patient can be seen by a clinician, be given a professional clinical judgment, and receive care that is ordered.

Discussion

This standard intends to ensure that juveniles have access to care to meet their serious health needs and is the principle on which all National Commission on Correctional Health Care standards are based. It is also the basic principle established by the U.S. Supreme Court in the 1976 landmark case *Estelle v. Gamble*.

Unreasonable barriers to juveniles' access to health services are to be avoided. Examples of unreasonable barriers include the following:

1. punishing juveniles for seeking care for their serious health needs;
2. assessing co-payments that prevent or deter juveniles from seeking care for their serious health needs;
3. deterring juveniles from seeking care for their serious health needs, such as holding sick call at 2 a.m., when this practice is not reasonably related to the needs of the facility;
4. permitting unreasonable delays before juveniles are seen by prescribing clinicians or outside consultants to obtain necessary diagnostic work or treatment for their serious health needs;
5. interfering with the prompt transmittal to health staff of a juvenile's oral or written request for care; or
6. preventing juveniles from attending sick call due to conflicts with school or work program schedules.

Optional Recommendation

The NCCHC position statement Charging Inmates a Fee for Health Care Services offers additional guidance about fee-for-service programs; it is available at www.ncchc.org. NCCHC requires that the use of such a fee-for-service program in a juvenile facility be reviewed closely as it generally would not be considered appropriate.

Y-A-02
essential

RESPONSIBLE HEALTH AUTHORITY

Standard

The facility has a designated health authority responsible for *health care* services.

Compliance Indicators

1. The responsible health authority (RHA) arranges for all levels of health care and assures quality, accessible, and timely health services for juveniles.
2. The RHA's responsibilities are documented in a written agreement, contract, or job description.
3. The RHA is on site at least weekly.
4. The RHA may be a physician, *health administrator*, or agency. Where the agency acting as RHA is a state, regional, corporate, or national entity, there is also a designated individual at the local level to ensure that policies are carried out.
5. Clinical judgments rest with a single, designated, licensed, *responsible physician*.
6. Where there is a separate organizational structure for mental health services, there is a *designated mental health clinician*.
7. All aspects of the standard are addressed by written policy and defined procedures.

Definitions

Health care is the sum of all actions, preventive and therapeutic, taken for the physical and mental well-being of a population. Health care includes medical, dental, mental health, nutrition, and other ancillary services, as well as maintaining clean and safe environmental conditions.

A *health administrator* is a person who by virtue of education, experience, or certification (e.g., MSN, MPH, MHA, FACHE, CCHP) is capable of assuming responsibility for arranging all levels of health care and ensuring quality and accessible health services for juveniles.

A *responsible physician* is a designated MD or DO who has the final authority at a given facility regarding clinical issues.

A *designated mental health clinician* refers to a psychiatrist, psychologist, or psychiatric social worker who is responsible for clinical mental health issues when mental health services at the facility are under a different authority than the medical services.

Qualified health care professionals include physicians, physician assistants, nurses, nurse practitioners, dentists, mental health professionals, and others who by virtue of their education, credentials, and experience are permitted by law to evaluate and care for patients.

Discussion

This standard seeks to ensure a coordinated health care system. The RHA functions to assure that health services are organized, adequate, and efficient. If this designated authority is not a physician, the responsible physician supervises the clinical aspects of health care.

The RHA implements corrective actions and monitors outcomes as a result of changes, adjusting and revising plans as needed. Such actions reflect an integrated health services program in which problems are identified through one process.

A single, designated responsible physician is required in all instances. The responsible physician supervises clinical judgments regarding the care provided to juveniles at the facility. This includes establishing and implementing policies for the clinical aspects of the program; monitoring the appropriateness, timeliness, and responsiveness of care and treatment; and reviewing the recommendations for treatment made by health care clinicians in the community.

Optional Recommendation

When a facility's satellite program is a significant distance from the main unit, it is recommended that an on-site *qualified health care professional* be designated as the RHA for the satellite. (See also Y-C-08 Health Care Liaison.)

Y-A-03
essential

MEDICAL AUTONOMY

Standard

Clinical decisions and actions regarding health care provided to juveniles to meet their serious medical needs are the sole responsibility of qualified health care professionals.

Compliance Indicators

1. Clinical decisions and their implementation are completed in an effective and safe manner.
2. Administrative decisions (such as utilization review) are coordinated, if necessary, with clinical needs so that patient care is not jeopardized.
3. *Child care staff* supports the implementation of clinical decisions.
4. *Health staff* is subject to the same security regulations as other facility employees.

5. All aspects of the standard are addressed by written policy and defined procedures.

Definitions

Child care staff includes line security as well as correctional administration.

Health staff includes all qualified health care professionals as well as administrative and support staff (e.g., health record administrators, laboratory technicians, nursing and medical assistants, clerical workers).

Discussion

The standard intends to ensure that clinical decisions are made for clinical purposes and without interference from other personnel.

The delivery of health care in a juvenile correctional facility is a joint effort of child care and health staffs and is best achieved through trust and cooperation. The responsible health authority arranges for the availability and monitoring of health care services. The official responsible for the facility provides the administrative support for the accessibility of health services to juveniles and the physical resources for the delivery of health care in a safe and professional manner.

The nonmedical considerations needed to carry out such clinical decisions are made in cooperation with child care staff. If this cooperation is lacking, such as when child care staff numbers are too low to carry out day-to-day medical support services, the ability of the health care professionals to perform their professional and legal responsibilities is impaired and medical autonomy is jeopardized. Other examples of interference by child care staff with medical autonomy include cancellation of scheduled community consultants' appointments and discontinuance of necessary medical diets during periods of sustained lockdown.

Specific problems that arise with medical autonomy generally are addressed through revised policies or reviewed as part of the continuous quality improvement program.

Y-A-04
essential

ADMINISTRATIVE MEETINGS AND REPORTS

Standard

Health (including oral and mental health) services are discussed at administrative meetings. In addition, health staff meetings are held to review administrative issues.

Compliance Indicators

1. Administrative meetings are attended by the facility administrator and the responsible health authority (RHA) or their designees, and other members of the health and child care staffs as appropriate. If mental health operates under a structure separate from other health services, the designated mental health clinician, or his or her designee, also attends.
2. Administrative meetings are held quarterly. Minutes or summaries are made and retained for reference, and copies are distributed to attendees.
3. Health staff meetings occur at least monthly and are documented.
4. Statistical reports of health services are made at least quarterly and provided to the facility administrator.
5. The number and types of statistics to be documented include, at a minimum:
   a. the number of juveniles receiving health services by category of care,
   b. referrals to specialists,
   c. deaths,
   d. infectious disease monitoring (e.g., hepatitis, HIV, sexually transmitted infections, tuberculosis),
   e. emergency services provided to patients, and
   f. dental procedures performed.
6. All aspects of the standard are addressed by written policy and defined procedures.

Discussion

This standard is intended to facilitate the health care delivery system through joint monitoring, planning, and problem resolution by the facility's health and correctional administrators. It is also intended that health staff are kept informed about facility operational issues.

Administrative meetings involve the RHA and the facility administrator, or their designees, and in facilities where mental health services are under separate authority, the designated mental health clinician. Topics of discussion include health care services, such as quality improvement findings (see Y-A-06 Continuous Quality Improvement Program), infection control efforts (see Y-B-01 Infection Control Program), inmate grievances (see Y-A-11 Grievance Mechanism for Health Complaints), and environmental inspection reports (see Y-B-02 Environmental Health and Safety).

Health staff meetings, held monthly or more frequently, give the health staff an opportunity to receive current information on all aspects of the facility's health care delivery. The meetings are documented in some fashion, either through formal minutes or, at a minimum, notations of when they were held and who attended, as well as an outline of the topics discussed.

Quarterly statistical reports are compiled and used to monitor trends in the delivery of health care. These include service volume; proportion of service types; and incidence of certain illnesses, diseases, and injuries targeted for risk management. These reports also are used to plan for staffing, space, and equipment needs, as well as to compare facilities.

Optional Recommendations

Minutes of administrative meetings should include an account of the effectiveness of the health care system, a description of any health environmental factor that may need improvement, changes made since the last report, and, if necessary, recommended corrective action.

Additional statistics that may be beneficial include the number of no-shows for health services, outside hospitalizations/services, physician on-site hours (including midlevel practitioner hours as a subcategory), dental services, mental health services, substance abuse services, and utilization of the infirmary.

It is recommended that other health staff attend when issues directly relating to their area of responsibility will be discussed (e.g., attendance by the responsible physician to discuss implementation of a vaccination program or by the dentist to discuss space needs in the dental area). When staff members are unable to attend health staff meetings, it is good practice for the RHA to obtain written confirmation that the vital information presented has been reviewed.

Health staff are encouraged to attend other facility staff meetings to promote good working relationships.

Y-A-05
essential

POLICIES AND PROCEDURES

Standard

There is a manual or compilation of written *policies* and defined *procedures* regarding health care services at the facility that addresses each applicable standard in the *Standards for Health Services in Juvenile Detention and Confinement Facilities*.

Compliance Indicators

1. Health care policies and procedures are site specific.
2. Each policy and procedure in the health care manual is reviewed at least annually, and revised as necessary under the direction of the responsible health authority (RHA). The manual bears the date of the most recent review or revision and, at a minimum, the signature of the facility's RHA and responsible physician.

3. Other policies, such as those for child care, kitchen, industries, or corporate, do not conflict with health care policies.
4. The manual or compilation is accessible to health staff.
5. All aspects of the standard are addressed by written policy and defined procedures.

Definitions

A *policy* is a facility's official position on a particular issue related to an organization's operations.

A *procedure* describes in detail, sometimes in sequence, how a policy is to be carried out.

Discussion

This standard intends to ensure that policies and procedures are written and available to staff. A policies and procedures manual is an important reference for new as well as established health staff.

A facility need not develop policies and procedures for standards that do not apply to it, such as Y-G-07 Care of the Pregnant Juvenile when females are not held at the facility or Y-G-03 Infirmary Care when the facility does not have an infirmary.

Some RHAs insert a signed and dated declaration at the beginning of the manual stating that policies and procedures have been reviewed and approved. Others require that each health services policy and procedure be signed by the RHA and responsible physician. Either is acceptable. However, when changes to individual health services policies are made, they must be dated and signed individually by the RHA and responsible physician.

This standard recognizes that all policies and procedures governing health services operations may not be promulgated by the same authority. For example, policies on child care staff training, recreational exercise, smoking, and personal hygiene often are promulgated by the child care worker administration rather than health services. It is not necessary for health services to write its own policy statements on such topics. Rather, the governing policies may be compiled as an addendum to the health services policy manual. Authorizing dates and signatures are required on all policies and procedures regardless of issuing authority, but those not promulgated by health services need not be signed by the RHA.

Annual review of policies, procedures, and programs is good management practice. This review facilitates incorporating changes made during the year into the facility's manual and encourages decisions about previously discussed but unresolved matters.

Optional Recommendation

Each policy should be cross-referenced with the relevant NCCHC standard or standards. However, it is not necessary that each standard have a separate policy and procedure statement (i.e., more than one standard may be addressed in the same policy and procedure, or several policies may address a single standard).

Y-A-06
essential

CONTINUOUS QUALITY IMPROVEMENT PROGRAM

Standard

A *continuous quality improvement (CQI) program* monitors and improves health care delivered in the facility.

Compliance Indicators

1. A CQI program identifies problems, implements and monitors corrective action, and studies its effectiveness.
2. The responsible physician is involved in the CQI program, e.g., by identifying thresholds, interpreting data, and solving problems.
3. Facilities with an average daily population (ADP) of 500 or less have a basic CQI program that:
   a. completes an annual review of the effectiveness of the CQI program by reviewing CQI studies, minutes of administrative and/or staff meetings, or other pertinent written materials; and
   b. performs at least one *process* quality improvement study and one *outcome* quality improvement study per year, where:
      i. a facility problem is identified,
      ii. a study is completed,
      iii. a plan is developed and implemented,
      iv. results are monitored and tracked, and
      v. improvement is demonstrated or the problem is restudied.
4. Facilities with an average daily population of greater than 500 juveniles have a comprehensive CQI program that does the following:
   a. establishes a *multidisciplinary quality improvement committee* that meets as required, but no less than quarterly, designs quality improvement monitoring activities, discusses the results, and implements corrective action;
   b. completes an annual review of the effectiveness of the CQI program by reviewing CQI studies and minutes of CQI, administrative, and/or staff meetings, or other pertinent written materials; and
   c. performs at least two *process* quality improvement studies and two *outcome* quality improvement studies per year, where:
      i. a facility problem is identified,
      ii. a study is completed,
      iii. a plan is developed and implemented,

iv.   results are monitored and tracked, and

v.   improvement is demonstrated or the problem is restudied.

5.   All aspects of the standard are addressed by written policy and defined procedures.

Definitions

The *basic CQI program* includes monitoring the fundamental aspects of the facility's health care system through one outcome study and one process study (e.g., access to care, the intake process, continuity of care, emergency care and hospitalizations, adverse patient occurrences including all deaths) at least annually.

The *comprehensive CQI program* includes a multidisciplinary quality improvement committee, monitoring of the areas specified in the compliance indicators, and an annual review of the effectiveness of the CQI program itself. In addition, the program includes two process quality improvement studies and two outcome quality improvement studies, and both studies identify areas in need of improvement and effect remedial actions or strategies.

A *multidisciplinary quality improvement committee* is a group of health staff from various disciplines (e.g., medicine, nursing, mental health, dentistry, health records, pharmacy, laboratory) that designs quality improvement monitoring activities, discusses the results, and implements corrective action.

Process quality improvement studies examine the effectiveness of the health care delivery process.

Outcome quality improvement studies examine whether expected outcomes of patient care were achieved.

Discussion

This standard is intended to ensure that a facility uses a structured process to find areas in the health care delivery system that need improvement, and that when such areas are found, staff develop and implement strategies for improvement.

Facilities with ADPs of fewer than 100 juveniles successfully apply basic CQI principles by focusing the annual review and the process and outcome quality improvement studies on issues and problems directly related to short-term admissions.

One essential element of quality improvement is the monitoring of high-risk, high-volume, or problem-prone aspects of health care provided to patients; however, not every aspect of every major service needs to be studied.

If established, a CQI committee meets at least quarterly to establish objective criteria for use in monitoring the quality of care, develop plans for improvement based on monitoring findings, and assess the effectiveness of these plans after implementation. If there is no CQI committee, this monitoring may be done as part of the administrative and/or staff meetings.

The responsible physician has a leadership role in the CQI process. Certain events, such as acute care hospital admissions, medical emergencies, and deaths, must be reviewed routinely.

Periodic reviews by outside groups such as public health departments and county medical societies undertaking peer review may be included in the quality improvement program but do not, by themselves, constitute compliance with this standard.

One of the benefits of a successful CQI program is that problems can be identified early and strategies developed for their resolution before they worsen.

Optional Recommendations

All health staff could benefit by receiving minutes or summaries of CQI activities.

Health staff responsible for guiding the CQI program should be given training opportunities to enhance their skills and the program's effectiveness.

CQI minutes should provide sufficient detail to guide future decisions. For example, the minutes could state the problems identified, the solutions that were agreed on, the person responsible for carrying out the corrective action, and the time frame for taking the corrective action.

CQI programs are more effective if they are inclusive. Representatives of child care staff should be involved as appropriate. Also, consideration should be given to conducting patient satisfaction surveys.

A systemwide (e.g., state, regional, corporate) CQI committee also may be established. Such a committee has representation from each facility and evidences two-way communication between the central CQI committee and facility health staff.

For further information, see Appendix C – Continuous Quality Improvement.

Y-A-07
essential

EMERGENCY RESPONSE PLAN

Standard

Health staff are prepared to implement the health aspects of the facility's emergency response plan.

Compliance Indicators

1. The health aspects of the emergency response plan are approved by the responsible health authority and facility administrator, and include at a minimum:
    a. responsibilities of health staff,
    b. procedures for triage,
    c. predetermination of the site for care,
    d. telephone numbers and procedures for calling health staff and the community emergency response system (e.g., hospitals, ambulances),
    e. procedures for evacuating patients, and
    f. alternate backups for each of the plan's elements.
2. At least one *mass disaster drill* and one *juvenile-down drill* are conducted annually in the facility.
3. The mass disaster and juvenile-down drills are *critiqued* and the results shared with all health staff.
4. If there are no full-time health staff at the facility, drills are not required.
5. All aspects of the standard are addressed by written policy and defined procedures.

Definitions

A *mass disaster drill* is a simulated emergency involving multiple casualties that require triage by health staff. It frequently involves a natural disaster (e.g., tornado, flood, earthquake), an internal disaster (e.g., riot, arson, kitchen explosion), or external disaster (e.g., mass arrests, bomb threat, power outage).

A *juvenile-down drill* is a simulated emergency affecting one individual who needs immediate medical intervention. It involves life-threatening situations commonly experienced in correctional settings.

Critiques of drills or actual events document activities including response time, names and titles of health staff, and the roles and responses of all participants. The critique contains observations of appropriate and inappropriate staff response to the drill.

Tabletop exercises are discussions about health staff's projected response to emergencies.

Discussion

This standard intends to ensure that a facility protects the health, safety, and welfare of juveniles, staff, and visitors during emergencies.

Emergency planning requires an appropriate health staff response including coordination with community emergency services, when necessary.

Practicing the emergency response plan makes health staff better able to respond to disasters when they occur. Drills also help to identify weaknesses in the facility's disaster plan. Although classroom or *tabletop exercises* can be useful, they are not sufficient to meet this standard. When actual emergencies, whether or not they involve injuries, are critiqued, the intent of this standard is met.

It is recognized that not all health staff on a particular shift may be present when a juvenile-down or mass disaster drill takes place. Staff members who are not present during a drill later review and initial the written critiques.

The mass disaster drill need not be practiced by all shifts each year; at a minimum, the drill is practiced once by each shift on a rotating basis over a 3-year period.

Fire drills with no simulated casualties do not meet the intent of the standard.

Optional Recommendations

It is recommended that where health staff are on duty on different shifts, each shift practices the health portions of a mass disaster drill. Since most emergencies are "juvenile-down" situations, facilities are encouraged to practice the annual health emergency juvenile-down drill on each shift where health staff are regularly assigned.

If case injuries need to be treated on site, separate emergency supplies should be stored and regularly checked.

Child care staff representatives should participate with health staff in planning and implementing mass disaster and juvenile-down drills. It also may be helpful for facility juveniles and community response agencies to participate in the drills.

Y-A-08
essential

COMMUNICATION ON PATIENTS WITH SPECIAL NEEDS

Standard

Communication occurs between the facility administration and treating health care professionals regarding juveniles' significant health needs that must be considered in classification decisions in order to preserve the health and safety of that juvenile, other juveniles, and staff.

Compliance Indicators

1. *Child care* staff are advised of juveniles' special needs that may affect housing, work, and program assignments; disciplinary measures; and admissions to and transfers from institutions. Such communication is documented.
2. Health and child care staff communicate about juveniles who are:
   a. *chronically ill,*
   b. on *dialysis,*
   c. infected with *serious communicable diseases,*
   d. *physically disabled,*
   e. pregnant,
   f. *frail,*
   g. *terminally ill,*
   h. mentally ill or suicidal,
   i. *developmentally disabled,* or
   j. vulnerable to abuse and manipulation.
3. All aspects of the standard are addressed by written policy and defined procedures.

Definitions

For definitions of conditions that result in special needs, see Y-G-02 Patients With Special Health Needs, Y-G-01 Chronic Disease Services, and the Glossary.

Discussion

This standard intends to ensure that child care staff are aware of the special needs and any restrictions they are to accommodate in making classification decisions.

Cooperation between child care personnel and health care professionals helps make both groups aware of juvenile movements and decisions regarding special needs patients. Medical or mental health problems may complicate housing assignments, work assignments, program assignments, disciplinary management (see Y-E-09 Segregated Juveniles), or transfers to another facility (see Y-E-10 Patient Escort).

In cases where the mental health and medical authorities are under different jurisdictions, the mental health clinician shares pertinent information with the facility administrator regarding juvenile mental health needs.

Y-A-09
important

PRIVACY OF CARE

Standard

Discussion of patient information and clinical encounters are conducted in private and carried out in a manner designed to encourage the patient's subsequent use of health services.

Compliance Indicators

1. *Clinical encounters* and discussions are conducted in private, without being observed or overheard.
2. At a minimum, verbal permission is obtained and consideration of gender-appropriate chaperone is made when a breast, rectal, pelvic, or external genitalia examination is indicated.
3. Child care personnel are present only if the patient poses a probable risk to the safety of the health care professionals or others.
4. Instruction on maintaining confidentiality is given to child care staff or interpreters who observe or hear health encounters.
5. All aspects of the standard are addressed by written policy and defined procedures.

Definition

Clinical encounters are interactions between patients and health care professionals that involve a treatment and/or an exchange of confidential information.

Discussion

The intent of this standard is to ensure that health care encounters and exchanges of information remain private and that a patient's dignity is protected. Such efforts foster necessary and candid conversation between patient and health care professional.

Arrangements should be made for an interpreter or other assistive devices when effective communication during the clinical encounter is compromised by deficits in speech or hearing, or the inability to communicate in the same language. Selection of the interpreter or form of assistance should consider the juvenile's communication preference and desire for privacy. Generally, the use of another juvenile as the interpreter should be limited to urgent situations.

Privacy is made more difficult when triaging health complaints at the juvenile's room or in segregated housing. When triage is required in the juvenile's room, health care professionals take extra precautions to promote private communication between health staff and the juvenile.

When safety is a concern and full privacy is lacking, it is recommended that alternative strategies for partial visual privacy, such as a privacy screen, or partial auditory privacy, such as white noise devices (to mask normal conversation) be considered.

Y-A-10
important

PROCEDURE IN THE EVENT OF A JUVENILE DEATH

Standard

All deaths are reviewed to determine the appropriateness of clinical care; to ascertain whether changes to policies, procedures, or practices are warranted; and to identify issues that require further study.

Compliance Indicators

1. All deaths are reviewed within 30 days.
2. A death review consists of:
   a. an *administrative review*,
   b. a *clinical mortality review*, and
   c. a *psychological autopsy* if death is by suicide.
3. Treating staff are informed of the clinical mortality review and administrative review findings.
4. Corrective actions identified through the mortality review process are implemented and monitored through the facility's continuous quality improvement program for systemic issues, and through the patient safety program for staff-related issues.
5. All aspects of the standard are addressed by written policy and defined procedures.

Definitions

An *administrative review* is an assessment of correctional and emergency response actions surrounding a juvenile's death. Its purpose is to identify areas where facility operations, policies, and procedures can be improved.

A *clinical mortality review* is an assessment of the clinical care provided and the circumstances leading up to a death. Its purpose is to identify areas of patient care or system policies and procedures that can be improved.

A *psychological autopsy*, sometimes referred to as a psychological reconstruction and usually conducted by a psychologist or other qualified mental health professional, is a written reconstruction of an individual's life with an emphasis on factors that may have contributed to the death.

Discussion

The intent of the standard is that preventable deaths are avoided.

A clinical mortality review is conducted to determine the appropriateness of the clinical care provided and the effectiveness of the facility's policies and procedures relevant to the circumstances surrounding the death. Generally, a clinical mortality review asks at least three key questions: Could the medical response at the time of death be improved? Was an earlier intervention possible? Independent of the cause of death, is there any way to improve patient care?

When multiple deaths occur at a facility, an assessment is done to determine whether any patterns require further study. The clinical mortality review is done separate and apart from other formal investigations that may be required to determine the cause of death.

The clinical mortality review may be conducted by a unit physician not involved in the patient's treatment, a central office or corporate physician, or an outside medical group. Regardless of who conducts the review, the results are to be communicated to the unit health staff involved.

The clinical mortality review includes a review of the incident and facility procedures used; training received by involved staff; pertinent medical and mental health services or reports involving the juvenile; and recommendations, if any, for change in policy, training, physical plant, medical or mental health services, and operational procedures. For expected deaths, a modified review process that focuses on the relevant clinical aspects of the death and preceding treatment may be followed.

Refer to Y-A-06 Continuous Quality Improvement Program and Y-B-03 Patient Safety for additional information and guidance.

When a medical autopsy is completed after the clinical mortality review is completed, the clinical review is appended with information from the autopsy report.

Included in the death review are those deaths, whether natural or otherwise, that occur off site while the facility is responsible for the juvenile.

Optional Recommendation

A postmortem examination can be very helpful and should be requested. The information can increase treating staff's understanding of the pathology of disease.

Y-A-11
important

GRIEVANCE MECHANISM FOR HEALTH COMPLAINTS

Standard

A grievance mechanism addresses juveniles' complaints about health services.

Compliance Indicators

1. The grievance policy includes a time frame for response and the process for appeal.
2. Responses to juvenile grievances are timely and based on principles of adequate medical care.
3. All aspects of the standard are addressed by written policy and defined procedures.

Discussion

A patient's right to question or complain about the health care system is protected.

Grievance mechanisms are an important component of a facility's quality improvement program (see Y-A-06 Continuous Quality Improvement Program). Well-founded grievances can provide health staff with valuable feedback regarding opportunities for improving health services. While not all complaints from juveniles are well-founded, those that are can help administrators identify problems with specific health care professionals or procedures. If someone other than a member of the health staff responds to grievances, health staff input is solicited before responding to a juvenile's health complaint.

Some facilities include health complaints in their formal grievance process while others have a separate procedure. Either method is acceptable.

Timeliness of the response to sick-call requests is an important indicator of quality of care and grievances should be tracked and analyzed through the continuous quality improvement process. High numbers of grievances or hospital emergency room visits may point to the need for increased physician time.

Optional Recommendations

Attempts should be made to informally resolve juveniles' complaints regarding health services. A face-to-face interview by a health services administrator, responsible physician, or nursing supervisor is often an effective way to resolve problems and demonstrate health staff's concern.

In addition, periodic dialogue with juvenile representatives regarding health service delivery issues is especially helpful in facilities with long-term populations. Such a practice is particularly useful in identifying and resolving systemic problems in health care delivery.

Y-A-12
important

NOTIFICATION IN EMERGENCIES

Standard

The facility notifies the juvenile's legal guardian in case of serious illness, injury, or death.

Compliance Indicators

1. When health staff become aware of the serious illness, injury, or death of a juvenile, health staff alert designated child care staff of the situation.
2. All aspects of the standard are addressed by written policy and defined procedures.

Discussion

The policy should specify when notification of the juvenile's legal guardian must occur (e.g., "any illness or injury resulting in hospitalization, and in all cases of death") and who is responsible for such notification (e.g., the facility administrator, a chaplain, a social worker, or the responsible physician).

SECTION B – SAFETY

Y-B-01
essential

INFECTION CONTROL PROGRAM

Standard

There is an effective infection control program.

Compliance Indicators

1. The responsible health authority (RHA) has a written *exposure control plan* that is approved by the responsible physician. The plan is reviewed and updated annually.
2. The RHA ensures that:
   a. medical, dental, and laboratory equipment and instruments are decontaminated properly;
   b. sharps and biohazardous wastes are disposed of properly;
   c. surveillance to detect juveniles with serious infectious and communicable disease is effective;
   d. immunizations to prevent disease are provided when appropriate;
   e. infected patients receive medically indicated care; and
   f. if appropriate, juveniles with contagious diseases are *medically isolated.*
3. When medical isolation is provided on site, juveniles should be checked frequently for changes in physical and mental status, and are accommodated in a separate room with:
   a. a separate toilet,
   b. hand-washing facility,
   c. soap dispenser, and
   d. single-service towels.
4. *Standard precautions* are always used by health care staff to minimize the risk of exposure to blood and body fluids of patients.
5. All sanitation workers are trained in proper methods for handling and disposing of biohazardous materials and spills.
6. If treated on site, active tuberculosis patients are housed in designated negative pressure rooms.
7. Juveniles who are released with communicable or infectious diseases are given community referrals.
8. The facility completes and files all reports as required by local, state, and federal laws and regulations.
9. Effective *ectoparasite* control procedures are used to treat infected juveniles and to disinfect bedding and clothing.
   a. Juveniles, bedding, and clothing infected with ectoparasites are disinfected.
   b. Prescribed treatment given to infected juveniles considers all conditions (such as pregnancy, open sores, or rashes) and is ordered only by clinicians.
   c. If the facility routinely delouses all juveniles, only over-the-counter medications, such as those containing pyrethrins, are used.

10. All aspects of the standard are addressed by written policy and defined procedures.

Definitions

An *exposure control plan* describes staff actions to be taken to eliminate or minimize exposures to pathogens.

Standard precautions combine the major features of universal precautions (designed to reduce the risk of transmission of bloodborne pathogens) and body secretion isolation (designed to reduce the transmission of pathogens from moist body substances) and apply them to all patients receiving care, regardless of their diagnosis or presumed infection status.

Ectoparasites such as pediculosis and scabies are parasites that live on the skin. They are communicable and may lead to secondary infections.

Discussion

The intent of this standard is to minimize the incidence of infectious and communicable diseases among juveniles.

Isolation practices include, but are not limited to, hand washing upon entering and exiting the patient's room; proper handling and disposal of infectious materials; proper isolation methods; instructions to the patient and to visitors; proper handling of food, utensils, and dishes; proper handling of patient care equipment; and cleaning and disinfecting of isolation housing areas. Further guidelines on ventilation, respiratory infection programs, and other infection control measures are available from the Centers for Disease Control and Prevention (CDC), the National Institute for Occupational Safety and Health (NIOSH), and the Occupational Safety and Health Administration (OSHA). Complete information about bloodborne exposure plans for infection control is also available from OSHA.

This standard is also intended to prevent harm to those being treated for ectoparasite infection. Screening for ectoparasites generally occurs at admission (see Y-E-02 Receiving Screening) and any time an outbreak occurs among juveniles who share living and bathroom facilities with an infected juvenile.

Optional Recommendations

In facilities with average daily populations of 150 or more, a committee (e.g., quality improvement, infection control) should oversee infection control practices. It is best to designate a single staff member as program coordinator. The infection control committee should have representation from the facility's administration, the responsible physician or designee, nursing and dental services, other appropriate professional personnel involved in sanitation or disease control, and the individual responsible for facility livestock or animals housed for programmatic purposes (e.g., dogs in training for guide duties), if appropriate. In a small facility, the physician or designee typically is responsible for the infection control program.

The facility should follow a tuberculosis control plan that is consistent with current published guidelines from the CDC.

Minimizing the number of needle injuries to health staff is important. Facilities are encouraged to have a needlestick prevention program that requires functional, accessible, and visible sharps disposal containers. Further guidance is available from relevant federal agencies and national organizations. Health staff also are encouraged to use needle safety devices such as self-sheathing needles or needle-less systems.

The use of a Wood's light can help to identify those infected with ectoparasites and can help to avoid the questionable practice of routinely delousing all juveniles.

Y-B-02
essential

ENVIRONMENTAL HEALTH AND SAFETY

Standard

The facility ensures that juveniles are housed, work, study, recreate, and receive health care in a clean, safe, and healthy environment.

Compliance Indicators

1. An environmental inspection of the facility is conducted at least monthly.
2. The monthly environmental inspection examines:
    a. the cleanliness and safety of juvenile housing, including segregation;
    b. laundry and housekeeping practices;
    c. pest control measures;
    d. risk exposure containment measures;
    e. equipment inspection and maintenance;
    f. occupational and environmental safety measures; and
    g. the cleanliness and sanitation of areas where health services are provided.
3. Written reports of the monthly inspections document corrective actions and are submitted to the facility administrator and responsible health authority (RHA).
4. All kitchen workers, including juveniles, are medically cleared and subsequently checked daily by supervising kitchen staff to ensure they are free from diarrhea, open sores, skin infections, and other illnesses transmissible by food or utensils.

5. Workers follow hygienic practices (e.g., washing hands before reporting to work, after touching contaminated surfaces, before preparing food, after using the toilet), and wear hairnets or caps when working with food.

6. Inspections of the kitchen, food storage, preparation, and dining areas are conducted at least monthly. There is evidence of corrective actions for negative findings.

7. All aspects of the standard are addressed by written policy and defined procedures.

Discussion

An intent of this standard is that the health of juveniles, staff, and visitors is protected through the maintenance of a clean and orderly facility.

A comprehensive environmental health program is important to the health and welfare of juveniles and staff (see Optional Recommendations below).

Another intent of this standard is to ensure a sanitary kitchen and proper food storage, handling, and preparation, all of which contribute to a healthy juvenile population. Food is protected from contamination and maintained at proper temperatures at all times, including when meals are transported to housing areas.

Medical clearance of food service workers before they begin working in the kitchen can be accomplished either through a review of the health record or a preservice physical examination.

The inspection of the kitchen, food storage, preparation, and handling areas confirms that areas are free of rodents and insects; floors, walls, and ceilings, as well as ducts, pipes, and equipment, are in good repair and free of particles (e.g., dirt, dust, dried food); traps and drains are free of standing water and debris; the gauges on dishwashing equipment, freezers, and refrigerators show temperatures in accordance with public health requirements; cooking and baking equipment, utensils, and food trays are washed, rinsed, and sanitized properly; food (raw and unprepared) is stored off the floor in closed containers, labeled with contents, and dated; and staff and juvenile worker bathrooms are in working order and have sinks, soap, paper supplies, and handwashing signs.

Optional Recommendations

Below are suggested components of the monthly inspection reports.

1. Juvenile housing. Each juvenile should be furnished with a single bed, clean mattress, pillow and case, sheets, blanket, and a locker or cabinet for the safe and orderly storage of personal property. There should be adequate lighting and noise containment. Hand-washing sinks, drinking fountains, showers, and toilets should be in sufficient numbers, accessible, with adequate water

pressure, clean, and in good repair. Hot water for showers should be thermostatically controlled at temperatures between 100 and 120 degrees.

2. Laundry. Laundry services, whether on site or contracted, should ensure the availability of a sufficient supply of clean linen and clothing. Each juvenile should be provided with daily changes of underwear and at least three clean changes of clothing, one clean change of bed linen, and three personal towels per week. Laundry of infectious or parasite-infected material is handled using precautions (e.g., gloves, gowns, masks) and properly bagged, labeled, and processed (see Y-F-04 Personal Hygiene).

3. Housekeeping. A comprehensive housekeeping program should identify what has to be cleaned, at what frequency, by whom, how it is to be cleaned, and who evaluates cleaning effectiveness and with what frequency. Sufficient and appropriate cleaning equipment and supplies, including water-soluble cleaning compounds, should be available for the housekeeping program. Refuse, including hazardous waste, should be handled, stored, and disposed of in a safe and sanitary manner consistent with local, state, and federal regulations.

4. Pest control. A pest control program should control the insect and rodent population. The pest control program should comply with federal and state laws.

5. Risk exposures. There should be a sufficient number of electrical outlets for the operation of equipment and appliances so that extension cords are used minimally. Fire retardation equipment (e.g., chemical tanks, fire hoses, air packs) should be kept in working order, and regular inspections of this equipment should be logged. Barber and beauty shops should be operated in conformance with applicable laws, rules, and regulations. Work areas sharing a common passage with sensitive service areas (e.g., dietary, commissary, laundry, health services) should have self-closing doors that are kept closed when not in use. Personal protective equipment (e.g., gloves, gowns, lab coats, face shields) should be available to all staff and juveniles who potentially may be exposed to infectious, parasitic, or hazardous materials or objects.

6. Equipment inspections. Regular inspections and servicing, consistent with manufacturer specifications and state regulations, should be undertaken for all heavy equipment (e.g., HVAC, generators, X-ray equipment, kitchen equipment) and operating systems (e.g., utilities, water supply, sewers) to ensure that all systems continue to function properly. Facility ventilation systems, especially negative pressure areas for the control of infectious disease, should be monitored regularly for air quality. See also standards Y-D-03 Clinic Space, Equipment, and Supplies and Y-D-04 Diagnostic Services.

7. Safety. All juveniles and staff are entitled to a safe and sanitary environment. Measures to ensure the safety of all who live, work, or visit within the facility should be undertaken as needed.

If an outbreak of a foodborne illness occurs, a sample of the food should be tested to identify the causative agent(s). Therefore, as a precaution, a sample of each meal served should be kept in the refrigerator for 24 hours (or longer as recommended by state authorities).

The RHA should consult local health department requirements for food service handlers (e.g., preservice physical examination, biomedical testing, special training).

Y-B-03
important

PATIENT SAFETY

Standard

The responsible health authority (RHA) promotes patient safety by instituting systems to prevent *adverse* and *near-miss* clinical events.

Compliance Indicators

1. The RHA proactively implements *patient safety systems* to prevent adverse and near-miss clinical events.
2. The RHA implements an *error reporting system* for health staff to voluntarily report, in a nonpunitive environment, errors that affect patient safety.
3. All aspects of the standard are addressed by written policy and defined procedures.

Definitions

An *adverse clinical event* is defined as an injury or death caused by medical management rather than by the patient's underlying disease or condition. A sizable proportion of adverse events in the community are the result of human errors. For example, switching two look-alike medications (e.g., Prozac and Doxipen) is a potentially easy mistake. Giving the wrong medication to patients during pill line administration is an adverse clinical event.

An *error reporting system* includes policies and procedures that outline how health staff voluntarily identify and report all clinical errors, whether the error occurs by omission (failing to do something that is supposed to be done) or commission (doing something that is not supposed to be done).

A *near-miss clinical event* is an error in clinical activity without a consequential adverse patient outcome. For example, a wrong drug is dispensed but not administered to a patient.

Patient safety systems are practice interventions designed to prevent adverse or near-miss clinical events. For example, during administration of medications, use of a photo identification system helps to ensure that the right person receives the right drug.

Discussion

The intent of this standard is to reduce risk and harm to patients. At a minimum, this includes health services leadership fostering a patient safety culture that encourages staff to identify opportunities to reduce harm or potential harm to patients. This can begin during staff orientation and training, and incorporate policies and procedures that guide staff in identifying and reporting potential problems.

A patient safety system focuses on strategies that improve clinical practice. For example, a patient safety system may include a stock medication bar-coding system, an ambulatory electronic prescription system, or a computerized care provider order entry system.

What is the difference between a patient safety system and a continuous quality improvement (CQI) program? CQI is a "process" approach to quality management that emphasizes the organization and system. CQI focuses on system issues rather than the individual and uses objective aggregate data to analyze and improve processes. The CQI process studies specific root causes and analyzes data to identify improvements in organizational structure and function. The CQI committee may study the patient safety system to determine needed improvements. Matters regarding individual clinical performance are generally not discussed in an open forum such as a CQI committee meeting.

In contrast, patient safety system problems are due to health professionals' action or inaction. Patient safety is proactive. For example, some facilities must rely on per diem workers, visiting health care professionals, or other temporary workers to augment their permanent staff. Maintaining access, confidentiality, and privacy of patient information is difficult under those circumstances. A patient safety program could include the use of an electronic medical record system to ensure that the facility complies with regulations and privacy requirements while facilitating clinical care.

Health care services provided in correctional facilities should promote patient safety in a nonpunitive, professional, and supportive environment. Health staff should be trained to promptly report unanticipated problems involving risk to patients. Issues relating to patient safety should be discussed during orientation and in-service training.

The RHA should analyze each adverse or near-miss clinical event. When the cause is due to a failure of policy or procedure, the CQI program should examine the issue. When at least part of the cause is due to individual competency, the RHA should initiate a process aimed at improving clinical skills or taking other appropriate action. For example, the RHA may perform a peer review, initiate a peer review by an outside practitioner, counsel the practitioner, require clinical supervision, require specific training, or offer employee assistance.

In most cases, affected patients should be informed when an adverse event has occurred. However, patient competency and the significance of the event may determine the appropriateness of disclosure.

The key to instilling a culture of patient safety is to understand that there is no one way to reduce error, no infallible system that prevents health staff from making errors. Rather, the health care administrator should employ a range of activities that communicate to staff that a culture of patient safety is a matter of attentiveness to what is being done (or not done) and a willingness to speak up about it.

(See also Y-A-06 Continuous Quality Improvement Program, Y-A-10 Procedure in the Event of a Juvenile Death, Y-C-02 Clinical Performance Enhancement, and Y-G-05 Suicide Prevention Program.)

Y-B-04
important

STAFF SAFETY

Standard

Health staff work in a safe environment.

Compliance Indicators

1. Measures to ensure the safety of health staff are undertaken.
2. All aspects of the standard are addressed by written policy and defined procedures.

Definition

Staff safety refers to the health and well-being of health staff who work in the facility. It is directly related to the administrative practice that ensures public safety of the facility.

Discussion

The intent of this standard is to reduce risk and harm to health staff.

The ability of health staff to provide health care is predicated on a safe and secure environment. Staff safety is more than sanitation and equipment checks. It also includes an environment where staff feel safe to do their work.

Y-B-05
important

FEDERAL SEXUAL ASSAULT REPORTING REGULATIONS

Standard

The facility has written policy and procedures regarding the detection, prevention, reduction, and punishment of rape consistent with federal law.

Compliance Indicator

All aspects of the standard are addressed by written policy and defined procedures.

Discussion

The intent of the standard is for correctional facilities to comply with applicable federal law. The *Prison Rape Elimination Act of 2003* addresses the many aspects of rape in correctional institutions, including the actions to be taken by correctional administrators, and is the foundation of this standard.

Y-B-06
important

PROCEDURE IN THE EVENT OF SEXUAL ASSAULT

Standard

The medical and psychological trauma of a *sexual assault* is minimized as much as possible by prompt and appropriate health intervention.

Compliance Indicators

1. Victims of sexual assault are either referred to a community facility for treatment and gathering of evidence, or if these procedures are performed in-house, the following guidelines are used.
   a. A history is taken and qualified health care professionals conduct an examination to document the extent of physical injury and to determine whether referral to another medical facility is indicated. With the victim's consent, the examination includes collection of evidence from the victim, using a kit approved by the local legal authority.
   b. Prophylactic treatment for sexually transmitted infections (e.g., HIV, hepatitis B), and follow-up care are offered to all victims, as appropriate. Emergency contraception is offered consistent with state law and the regulations of the jurisdiction.
   c. After the physical examination, there is an evaluation by a qualified mental health professional for crisis intervention counseling and long-term follow-up.
   d. A report is made to the correctional authorities to effect a separation of the victim from the assailant in their housing assignments.

2. Assessment of the adolescent victim for potential for suicide, anxiety disorders or other mental health problems is done.
3. All aspects of the standard are addressed by written policy and defined procedures.

Definition

A *sexual assault* is a sexual act that is coercive or assaultive in nature and involves the use or the threat of force.

Discussion

The standard intends that appropriate treatment takes place for victims of sexual assault.

Reports as required by law are filed with police agencies and child protective services of the jurisdiction. With the sexual assault victim's consent, health professionals are permitted to gather forensic evidence from the victim, even though, under this standard, they are not permitted to gather forensic evidence from the alleged perpetrator. However, medical information may be obtained from the alleged perpetrator, with his or her consent, so that appropriate medical intervention can be initiated for the victim.

Optional Recommendations

Immediate response to an act of sexual assault is of the utmost importance. Separation of the victim and alleged assailant is needed to protect the victim and to prevent further violence.

Psychological trauma may occur to individuals other than the victim of a sexual assault. Mental health staff should be available to provide support and assistance to those in need. Sexual assault is especially traumatic to adolescents; therefore, when an adolescent is the victim of sexual assault, the potential for suicide should be carefully assessed.

SECTION C – PERSONNEL AND TRAINING

Y-C-01
essential

CREDENTIALING

Standard

All health care personnel who provide services to juveniles are appropriately credentialed according to the licensure, certification, and registration requirements of the jurisdiction.

Compliance Indicators

1. The responsible health authority (RHA) assures that new hires undergo a credentialing verification process that confirms current licensure, certification, or registration.
2. The credentialing process includes inquiry regarding sanctions or disciplinary actions of state boards, employers, and the National Practitioner Data Bank (NPDB).
3. Health professionals do not perform tasks beyond those permitted by their credentials.
4. The RHA maintains verification of current credentials for all qualified health care professionals at a readily accessible location.
5. A license that restricts practice to correctional institutions is not in compliance with this standard.
6. All aspects of the standard are addressed by written policy and defined procedures.

Definition

Restricted licenses refers to licenses that have attached stipulations that must be followed. Different state licensing boards refer to these modified licenses by various names including temporary, probation, stipulated order or agreement, practice restriction, institutional, restricted, disciplinary, provisional, limited, and conditional.

Discussion

An intent of this standard is that the facility's qualified health care professionals are legally qualified.

It is the responsibility of health professionals to maintain their license, certification, or registration. It is helpful for the RHA to keep copies of these documents on site.

Procedures for verification of credentials of new hires should include the following: identification of the person responsible for conducting the verification; actions that person should take in the confirmation process; agencies that should be called; inquiries about sanctions or disciplinary actions that state boards, other employers, and the NPDB have taken; and procedures for periodic reconfirmation. Background checks for child and sexual abuse are required by law in some states.

Also see Y-C-02 Clinical Performance Enhancement.

Students in the various health professions may receive training in correctional environments to supplement services under the supervision of appropriate qualified health care professionals just as they would in a community setting. If used, students are properly oriented (see Y-C-09 Orientation for Health Staff) and identified. They do not perform tasks beyond those permitted by their student status.

Most facilities employ health care professionals qualified to work in a community setting as well as in the facility. There are some circumstances in which facilities may employ health professionals with restricted or probationary licenses; however, they may not employ so many that supervision, patient advocacy, or independent medical practice is compromised. (See the NCCHC position statement on Licensed Health Care Providers in Correctional Institutions, available at www.ncchc.org.)

Except for federal employees, licenses and credentials for health professionals are from the state in which they practice.

Y-C-02
important

CLINICAL PERFORMANCE ENHANCEMENT

Standard

A clinical performance enhancement process evaluates the appropriateness of all primary care clinicians' services.

Compliance Indicators

1. The clinical performance of the facility's *primary care clinicians* is reviewed at least annually.
2. *Clinical performance enhancement* reviews are kept confidential and incorporate at least the following elements: the name of the individual being reviewed, the date of the review, the name and credentials of the reviewer, confirmation that the review was shared with the clinician, and a summary of the findings and corrective action, if any.
3. A log or other written record providing the names of the primary care clinicians and the dates of their most recent reviews is available.
4. The responsible health authority (RHA) implements an *independent review* when there is serious concern about a health care clinician's competence.
5. The RHA implements procedures to improve a health care clinician's competence when such action is necessary.

6. All aspects of the standard are addressed by written policy and defined procedures.

Definitions

Clinical performance enhancement is the process of having a health professional's work reviewed by another professional of at least equal training in the same general discipline, such as the review of the facility's physicians by the responsible physician.

Primary care clinicians are all licensed practitioners providing the facility's *primary care;* this includes medical physicians, psychiatrists, dentists, midlevel practitioners (i.e., nurse practitioners, physician assistants), and PhD-level psychologists.

Primary care, according to the National Academy of Sciences' Institute of Medicine, is the provision of integrated, accessible health care services by clinicians who are accountable for addressing a large majority of personal health care needs, developing a sustained partnership with patients, and practicing in the context of family and community.

Independent review is the assessment of a health care professional's compliance with discipline-specific and community standards. The review includes an analysis of trends in a practitioner's clinical practice. This review may be conducted by someone who may or may not be directly employed by the facility, as long as the reviewing practitioner has not been previously involved in the care of the patient(s) involved.

Discussion

The intent of this standard is to enhance patient care through peer review of the clinicians' practice. The clinical performance enhancement review process is neither an annual performance review nor a clinical case conference process. It is a professional practice review focused on the practitioner's clinical skills; its purpose is to enhance competence and address areas in need of improvement. Results of clinical performance enhancement reviews are confidentially communicated to the reviewed clinician along with any recommendations. Appropriate follow-up or corrective action is undertaken as needed.

In large facilities, supervisors generally review the clinical care of other practitioners within their discipline. If the supervisors also provide clinical care, they also are reviewed through this process. Reviews may be accomplished through a memorandum of agreement with an outside practitioner, by contracting with an outside group (e.g., medical school, hospital), or through the regional or corporate system. A sponsoring or supervising physician or a peer midlevel practitioner may review the work of midlevel practitioners.

Optional Recommendation

A standardized review form is recommended.

Y-C-03
essential

PROFESSIONAL DEVELOPMENT

Standard

All qualified health care professionals participate annually in continuing education appropriate for their positions.

Compliance Indicators

1. Full-time qualified health care professionals obtain 12 hours of continuing education per year.
2. Part-time qualified health care professionals prorate their continuing education hours based on full-time equivalency.
3. Compliance can be demonstrated through one of the following options:
   a. In states where at least 12 hours of continuing education is required annually to maintain a clinical license to practice, a current license suffices.
   b. When the health staff is a Certified Correctional Health Professional (CCHP), valid certification suffices.
   c. A list of completed courses, dates, and number of hours per course are on file.
4. All qualified health care professionals who have patient contact are current in cardiopulmonary resuscitation technique.
5. All aspects of the standard are addressed by written policy and defined procedures.

Discussion

The standard intends that the facility's qualified health care professionals are kept current in clinical knowledge and skills.

Cardiopulmonary resuscitation training may be provided by an approved body, such as the American Red Cross or American Heart Association, or from an individual possessing a current instructor's certificate from an approved body.

Continuing education may include staff development experiences; instruction given on site by a member of the health staff or a guest lecturer; attendance at programs offered by the facility or in the community by universities, hospitals, or other health care professionals; or participation in programs such as NCCHC's conferences where formal continuing education credits are offered. Although self-study guides or review of Internet resources may be part of the facility's continuing education program, they may not constitute the whole program.

Optional Recommendations

In-service programs or attendance at conferences focusing on topics related to correctional health care are beneficial for health staff working in correctional settings. Presentations on the special health needs of adolescents should be included as topics for periodic in-service.

Y-C-04
essential

HEALTH TRAINING FOR CHILD CARE STAFF

Standard

A training program, established or approved by the responsible health authority in cooperation with the facility administrator, guides the health-related training of all child care staff who work with juveniles.

Compliance Indicators

1. Child care staff who work with juveniles receive health-related training at least every 2 years; at a minimum, this includes:
   a. administration of first aid,
   b. recognizing the need for emergency care and intervention in life-threatening situations (e.g., heart attack);
   c. recognizing acute manifestations of certain chronic illnesses (e.g., asthma, seizures), intoxication and withdrawal, and adverse reactions to medications;
   d. recognizing signs and symptoms of mental illness;
   e. procedures for suicide prevention;
   f. procedures for appropriate referral of juveniles with health complaints to health staff;
   g. precautions and procedures with respect to infectious and communicable diseases; and
   h. cardiopulmonary resuscitation.
2. The appropriateness of the health-related training is verified by an outline of the course content and the length of the course.
3. A certificate or other evidence of attendance is kept on site for each employee.
4. Child care workers assigned to outside programs (e.g., Outward Bound programs, forestry camps, or routine outdoor recreation) are current in CPR, first-aid training, and prevention of heat-related illness.
5. While it is expected that 100% of the child care staff who work with juveniles are trained in all of these areas, compliance with the standard requires that at least 85% of the staff present on each shift are current in their health-related training.
6. All aspects of the standard are addressed by written policy and defined procedures.

Discussion

This standard intends to promote the training of child care workers to recognize when the need to refer a juvenile to a qualified health care professional occurs and to provide emergency care until he or she arrives.

Because child care workers are often the first to respond to problems, they must be aware of the potential for emergencies that may arise, know the proper response to life-threatening situations, and understand their part in the early detection of illness and injury.

Optional Recommendation

Mental health staff should review the training curriculum to advise on its content regarding suicide prevention procedures, recognizing the signs and symptoms of mental illness and substance abuse, and communication skills for managing juveniles with mental disorders.

Y-C-05
essential

MEDICATION ADMINISTRATION TRAINING

Standard

Personnel who administer or deliver prescription medication are appropriately trained.

Compliance Indicators

1. Child care workers or health staff who administer or deliver prescription medication to juveniles are permitted by state law to do so and are trained as needed in matters of security, accountability, common side effects, and documentation of administration of medicines (see Y-D-01 Pharmaceutical Operations).
2. The training is approved by the responsible physician and facility administrator or designee.
3. Documentation of completed training and testing is kept on file for staff who administer or deliver medications.
4. All aspects of the standard are addressed by written policy and defined procedures.

Discussion

The intent of this standard is to ensure that prescription medications are properly administered. This helps to protect the patient's health, ensuring that the right drug is administered at the right time in the right dose by the right method to the right person. It is best to have medications administered by qualified health care professionals who have been appropriately trained to administer them.

Optional Recommendations

Training in the security aspects of medication administration should be given periodically to all staff involved. It is recommended that the training be conducted by qualified health care professionals and include posttraining evaluation.

Psychiatric staff should review the training materials to assess their content relating to the security, accountability, common side effects, and documentation of the administration of psychotropic medications.

Other issues that should be discussed during the medication administration and delivery training are hoarding of medications, selling of drugs, overdoses, and adherence to therapeutic regimens.

It is preferable that in facilities where health staff are on site 7 days a week for at least two shifts, qualified health care professionals administer the medications.

Y-C-06
essential

JUVENILE WORKERS

Standard

Juveniles involved in health services are appropriately trained and supervised.

Compliance Indicators

1. Juveniles do not make treatment decisions or provide patient care.
2. Juveniles do not distribute or collect sick-call slips, schedule appointments, or handle health records, medications, or surgical instruments and sharps.
3. Juveniles employed in cleaning the health services unit are appropriately trained and continuously supervised regarding their work assignments. Documentation of such training is maintained at the facility.
4. Juveniles are not substitutes for regular program staff, but may be involved in appropriate peer health-related programs.
5. All aspects of the standard are addressed by written policy and defined procedures.

Definition

Activities of daily living (ADL) generally refers to ambulation, bathing, dressing, feeding, and toileting.

Discussion

An intent of this standard is that the health services program is not used as a vehicle that places juveniles in a position of power over their peers. Understaffed correctional facilities may be tempted to use juveniles in health care delivery to perform services for which civilian personnel are not available. Their use frequently violates state laws, invites litigation, brings discredit to the correctional health care field, and gives juveniles unwarranted power over their peers.

It is recommended that juveniles not be permitted to provide janitorial services in the health services area. However, if juveniles clean the health services area, they are supervised closely and directly in areas that hold health records, medications, syringes, needles, sharp instruments, or supplies. When juveniles handle biohazardous waste, they may do so only after receiving appropriate training including use of protective materials. Training and protective materials for juvenile workers involved in handling biohazardous waste should adhere to Occupational Safety and Health Administration guidelines.

The use of juveniles in appropriate peer health-related programs is permitted. For example, juveniles may assist other juveniles in *activities of daily living* (ADL) in regular housing units. Juveniles also may participate in support groups. Juveniles are not used as substitutes for regular program or health staff.

Y-C-07
important

STAFFING

Standard

A sufficient number of health staff of varying types provide juveniles with adequate and timely evaluation and treatment consistent with contemporary standards of care.

Compliance Indicators

1. The responsible health authority approves the *staffing plan*.
2. The adequacy and effectiveness of the staffing plan are assessed by the facility's ability to meet the health needs of the juvenile population.
3. All aspects of the standard are addressed by written policy and defined procedures.

Definitions

A *staffing plan* lays out the full-time equivalent (FTE) staff coverage required, lists current incumbents and vacancies, and addresses how full coverage will be accomplished if all positions are not filled (e.g., use of agency, temporary, or part-time staff). A staffing plan is a detailed schedule on which classifications of staff are assigned to *posts* and *positions* for the health care unit.

A *post* is a job defined by its location, time, and duties that can be filled interchangeably by different staff members (e.g., 7-3 infirmary nurse). Continuous coverage usually distinguishes a post from a position; a post has tasks that cannot usually be deferred.

A *position* is a job filled by a specific staff member (e.g., medical records secretary, physician, chief nurse). A position has tasks that can usually be deferred until the staff member is available.

A *prescribing clinician* is a licensed individual, such as an MD, DO, NP, or PA, authorized to write prescriptions.

Discussion

An intent of this standard is that the health care delivery system has sufficient numbers and types of health staff to care for the juvenile population.

The number and types of qualified health care professionals required depend on the size of the facility, the types (e.g., medical, nursing, dental, mental health) and scope (e.g., outpatient, specialty care, inpatient care) of health services delivered, the needs of the juvenile population, and the organizational structure (e.g., hours of service, use of assistants, scheduling). Consideration is given to labor-intensive activities when developing a staffing plan. Such activities include medication distribution, sick call, and room checks in segregated housing. These and other factors are to be reflected in the staffing plan.

Volunteers and students are not included in the staffing plan for delivering basic health services.

While it is not possible to specify exact clinician-to-patient ratios, the amount of *prescribing clinician* time must be sufficient to ensure that there is no unreasonable delay in patients receiving necessary care.

The sufficiency of the staffing plan can be assessed by a number of factors. These include having an adequate number of physicians, midlevel practitioners, and support staff to provide necessary care, having timely and thorough physician encounters, and the length of the list of those waiting to be seen by the physician or other health care professionals.

Physician time must be sufficient to fulfill both clinical and administrative responsibilities. Clinical duties include, but are not limited to, conducting physical examinations, evaluating and managing patients in clinics, monitoring other clinicians by reviewing and cosigning charts, reviewing laboratory and other diagnostic test results, and developing individual treatment plans. Administrative responsibilities include, but are not limited to, reviewing and approving policies, procedures, protocols, and guidelines; participating in staff meetings; conducting in-service training programs; and participating in continuous quality improvement and infection control programs.

Where permitted by state law, nurse practitioners or physician assistants under the supervision of a physician can substitute for a portion of the physician's time seeing patients.

Y-C-08
essential

HEALTH CARE LIAISON

Standard

A designated, trained *health care liaison* coordinates the health delivery services in the facility when qualified health care professionals are not on site.

Compliance Indicators

1. The health care liaison is trained by, and under the joint supervision of, the responsible physician and the facility administrator or their designee.
2. Duties assigned to the health care liaison post are appropriately carried out.
3. All aspects of the standard are addressed by written policy and defined procedures.

Definition

The *health care liaison* generally carries out the following duties: reviewing receiving screening forms for follow-up attention; triaging nonemergency sick-call requests every 24 hours; facilitating sick call by having juveniles and records available for the health care professional; and helping to carry out clinicians' orders regarding such matters as diet, housing, and work assignments. The health care liaison may be a child care worker or other person without a health care license who is trained by the responsible physician in limited aspects of health care coordination.

Discussion

An intent of this standard is that juveniles continue to have access to health services when qualified health care professionals are not on site.

The need for a health care liaison depends on the availability of qualified health care professionals. On shifts where qualified health care professionals are not on duty, health care liaisons may communicate the health needs of juveniles to the responsible health authority.

Protocols guide health care liaisons. These protocols are approved by the responsible physician and give direction about the triaging of nonemergency sick-call requests. Training topics for the health care liaison include documentation, communication, and confidentiality of juveniles' health information.

Y-C-09
important

ORIENTATION FOR HEALTH STAFF

Standard

All health staff receive an immediate *basic orientation* and all full-time staff complete a formal *in-depth orientation* to the health services program.

Compliance Indicators

1. The orientation program is approved by the responsible health authority and the facility administrator.
2. The orientation lesson plan is reviewed once every 2 years or more frequently, as needed.
3. All health staff receive a basic orientation on the first day of on-site service and prior to patient contact. At a minimum, this addresses relevant security and health services policies and procedures, response to facility emergency situations, the staff member's functional position description, and juvenile-staff relationships.
4. Within 90 days of employment, all full-time health staff complete an in-depth orientation. At a minimum, this includes all health services policies and procedures not addressed in the basic orientation, health and age-specific needs of the juvenile population, infection control including use of standard precautions, and confidentiality of records and health information. The content may vary depending on the roles and responsibilities of the new staff member.
5. Completion of the orientation program is documented and kept on file.
6. All aspects of the standard are addressed by written policy and defined procedures.

Definitions

Basic orientation, which is provided on the first day of employment, includes information necessary for the health staff member (e.g., full-time, part-time, consultant, per diem) to function safely in the facility.

In-depth orientation includes a full familiarization with the health services delivery system at the facility, and focuses on the similarities and differences between providing health care in the community and in a correctional setting.

Discussion

This standard intends that health staff are properly acclimated to work in the correctional environment and understand their roles and responsibilities.

Providing health services in a correctional setting is a unique task that requires special orientation for personnel new to a facility or to corrections.

Although some systems require health staff to participate in an orientation to the custody environment at the facility or at a training academy, this does not substitute for the necessary basic and in-depth orientations to the health services delivery system at the facility.

Optional Recommendations

Additional topics that could be included in the formal orientation program are as follows: security, including classification; health care needs of the juvenile population; the juvenile social system; the organization of health services at the facility; and infection control. If the orientation program includes representatives from both the health and child care staffs, the special working relationship between the two can be demonstrated.

Orientation topics for nursing could also include assessment and sick-call triage, emergency triage and management, resource utilization outside the facility, procedures for release of information, expected documentation practices, isolation procedures, and professional boundaries.

Evaluation of the effectiveness of the orientation program should be part of the continuous quality improvement program. The use of an orientation checklist is usually helpful.

SECTION D – HEALTH CARE SERVICES AND SUPPORT

Y-D-01
essential

PHARMACEUTICAL OPERATIONS

Standard

Pharmaceutical operations are sufficient to meet the needs of the facility and are in accordance with legal requirements.

Compliance Indicators

1. The facility complies with all applicable state and federal regulations regarding prescribing, *dispensing, administering*, and *procuring* pharmaceuticals.
2. The facility maintains a *formulary* for clinicians.
3. The facility maintains procedures for the timely procurement, dispensing, *distribution, accounting*, and *disposal* of pharmaceuticals.
4. The facility maintains records as necessary to ensure adequate control of and accountability for all medications.
5. The facility maintains maximum security storage of, and accountability by use for, Drug Enforcement Agency *(DEA)-controlled substances*.
6. There is an adequate method for notifying the responsible practitioner of the impending expiration of a drug order so that the practitioner can determine whether the drug administration is to be continued or altered.
7. Medications are kept under the control of appropriate staff members.
8. Juveniles do not prepare, dispense, or administer medication except for *self-medication programs* approved by the facility administrator and responsible physician (e.g., keep-on-person programs). Juveniles are permitted to carry medications necessary for the emergency management of a condition when ordered by a clinician.
9. Drug storage and medication areas are devoid of outdated, discontinued, or recalled medications.
10. Where there is no staff pharmacist, a consulting pharmacist is used for documented inspections and consultation on a regular basis, not less than quarterly. All off-site locations are included in the inspection schedules.
11. All medications are stored under proper conditions of sanitation, temperature, light, moisture, ventilation, segregation, and security. Antiseptics, other medications for external use, and disinfectants are stored separately from internal and injectable medications. Medications requiring special storage for stability (e.g., medications that need refrigeration) are so stored.
12. An adequate and proper supply of antidotes and other emergency medications, and related information are readily available to the staff (including posting of the poison control telephone number in areas where overdoses or toxicologic emergencies are likely).
13. All aspects of the standard are addressed by written policy and defined procedures.

Definitions

Dispensing is the placing of one or more doses of a prescribed medication into containers that are correctly labeled to indicate the name of the patient, the contents of the container, and all other vital information.

Administering medication is the act in which a single dose of an identified drug is given to a patient.

Procuring is the act of ordering medications for the facility.

A *formulary* is a written list of prescription and nonprescription medications that are ordinarily available to authorized prescribers, including consultants, working for the facility.

Distribution is the system for delivering, storing, and accounting for medications from the source of supply to the nursing station or point where they are administered to the patient.

Accounting is the act of recording, summarizing, analyzing, verifying, and reporting medication usage.

Disposal is (a) the destruction of medication on its expiration date or when retention is no longer necessary or suitable (e.g., upon patient discharge from the facility), or (b) the provision of medication to the juvenile upon discharge from the facility (in accordance with the continuity-of-care principle).

DEA-controlled substances are the medications that come under the jurisdiction of the Federal Controlled Substances Act.

Self-medication programs (also known as keep-on-person programs) permit responsible juveniles to carry and administer their own medications.

Discussion

The intent of this standard is that the facility's pharmaceutical services are legally and properly operated.

A formulary usually is developed by the responsible physician and responsible health authority with the assistance of a consulting pharmacist or pharmacy and/or a pharmacy therapeutics committee. An exception procedure that enables the use of nonformulary medications when medically appropriate should also be developed.

Small facilities, or those using outside pharmacies, may use the current American Society of Health-System Pharmacists (ASHP) drug formulary for their reference list (i.e., Principles of a Sound Drug Formulary System and ASHP Guidelines on the Pharmacy and Therapeutics Committee and the Formulary System). The use of a formulary does not restrict prescriptions of medication generated by outside community health care professionals; however, these are still subject to review and approval by the responsible physician.

Facilities with on-site opioid treatment program (OTP) services that use methadone must comply with federal regulations (see NCCHC's *Standards for Opioid Treatment Programs in Correctional Settings*). Facilities using methadone for purposes other than detoxification or maintenance or those using community-based OTP programs do not require federal review.

Optional Recommendations

When a facility uses a sealed, prepackaged unit dose system, the unused portion should be returned to the pharmacy. When pharmacies will not accept returned medications or will accept them only to destroy them without a credit to the facility, the RHA might consider giving any unused portion of medication to the parent or guardian of the discharged juvenile for completion of prescribed therapy even if the amount is greater than the usual discharge medication provided.

Y-D-02
essential

MEDICATION SERVICES

Standard

Medication services are clinically appropriate and provided in a timely, safe, and sufficient manner.

Compliance Indicators

1. Prescription medications are administered or delivered to the patient only on the order of a physician, dentist, or other legally authorized individual.
2. The responsible physician determines prescriptive practices in the facility.
3. Medications are prescribed only when clinically indicated (e.g., psychotropic and behavior-modifying medications are not used for disciplinary purposes).
4. There is a procedure for identifying and correcting *medication errors.*
5. Juveniles entering the facility on prescription medication continue to receive the medication in a timely fashion as prescribed, or acceptable alternate medications are provided as clinically indicated.
6. All aspects of the standard are addressed by written policy and defined procedures.

Definition

Medication errors include errors of commission (wrong medication to patient, wrong dose of medication to patient, wrong schedule for medication, and wrong method of administration) and omission (prescribed medication not given).

Discussion

This standard intends that medication practices are commensurate with current community practice.

The responsible physician establishes the policies regarding all prescription medications administered or delivered in the facility. If a self-medication program is used, it is developed through collaboration and agreement between the facility administrator and responsible physician. The responsible physician develops a list of self-administered medications and related procedures in collaboration with the pharmacist.

A self-medication program can be beneficial, particularly if it includes patient education and monitoring. Patients learn to take more responsibility for their own health care. The program also can save staff time in administering medications and escorting patients to and from the clinic area. However, care needs to be taken to ensure the policies are specific as to who may participate, what medications may be included, and under what conditions the program is implemented. Juveniles who have diabetes or asthma, for example, need to be educated on how to handle their health needs, especially as the time for discharge approaches.

Clinicians should use psychotropic medications for incarcerated juveniles only in a safe and clinically appropriate manner and only as part of a comprehensive treatment plan.

Additional certification and accreditation may be required for opioid treatment. Clinicians prescribing the opioid agonist treatment medication buprenorphine should be certified to do so.

Unless medications are taken as prescribed, maintaining a therapeutic dose of medications may not be possible, which may have grave consequences to patient health. Juveniles being admitted who report taking medications currently or who bring the medications with them are to continue their medication unless there is a clinical reason to alter or discontinue the medication. Protocols are in place so that the drugs are administered in a timely fashion as dictated by clinical need.

In all medication service practices, adverse patient outcomes can occur when (1) the clinician frequently changes orders, (2) the clinician fails to review patient medication histories, or (3) treating clinicians are unaware of each other's prescribing practices (which also can encourage inappropriate juvenile drug-seeking behavior). Medication errors, whether there are adverse consequences or not, are the single most preventable cause of patient injury.

Optional Recommendations

The responsible physician has several options to ensure that juveniles admitted on prescribed medication continue to receive the necessary drugs in a timely manner. One protocol requires the physician or physician on-call to be contacted for a verbal order after health staff have verified the medication prescription by contacting the community prescribing clinician or pharmacy. Another authorizes the nurses to give the medications based on the community clinician's valid order until the facility physician can see the juvenile. Some protocols allow the use of medication brought into the facility if it comes in original pharmacy packaging, is labeled as required, and staff verify the order with the community prescriber or pharmacist.

Over-the-counter (OTC) medications received by juveniles from other than health staff (e.g., through the commissary) need not be documented in the health record. Administration of OTC medications by health staff, however, should be documented in the medication administration record.

The facility can use its continuous quality improvement program to focus periodically on these issues.

Health and child care staff should be aware of the potential phototoxic effects of medications (particularly psychotropics and acne medication). Patients taking these medications and exposed to sunlight should be provided with appropriate sunscreen or shading.

Y-D-03
important

CLINIC SPACE, EQUIPMENT, AND SUPPLIES

Standard

Sufficient and suitable space, supplies, and equipment are available for the facility's medical, dental, and mental health care services.

Compliance Indicators

1. Examination and treatment rooms for medical, dental, and mental health care are large enough to accommodate the necessary equipment, supplies, and fixtures, and to permit privacy during clinical encounters.
2. Pharmaceuticals, medical supplies, and mobile emergency equipment are available and checked regularly.
3. There is adequate office space with administrative files, secure storage of health records, and writing desks.

4. Mental health services are provided in an area with private interview space for both individual assessment and group treatment, as well as desks, chairs, lockable file space, and relevant testing materials.

5. When laboratory, radiological, or other ancillary services are provided on site, the designated area is adequate to hold equipment and records.

6. When patients are placed in a waiting area for more than a brief period, the waiting area has seats and access to drinking water and toilets.

7. At a minimum, daily inventories are maintained on items subject to abuse (e.g., syringes, needles, scissors, other sharp instruments).

8. If treatment and examinations take place on site (as opposed to a community medical setting), the facility has, at a minimum, the following equipment, supplies, and materials:
   a. hand-washing facilities or appropriate alternate means of hand sanitization,
   b. examination tables,
   c. a light capable of providing direct illumination, and
   d. trash containers for biohazardous materials and sharps.

9. All aspects of the standard are addressed by written policy and defined procedures.

Discussion

An intent of this standard is that the facility provides sufficient equipment and space to support the health services program. The amount of space and the configuration of the room(s) needed for the care and treatment of patients may vary with the size of the facility and the kinds of services provided on site.

The types of equipment, supplies, and materials for examination and treatment depend on the level of health care provided in the facility and the capabilities and needs of specific health care professionals.

The daily monitoring of sharps can be in the form of verification of the accuracy of daily logs or other types of monitoring systems.

In addition to equipment required by compliance indicator #8, the facility should have, at a minimum, the following equipment, supplies, and materials for the examination and treatment of patients:
   a. scales,
   b. thermometers,
   c. blood pressure monitoring equipment,
   d. stethoscope,
   e. ophthalmoscope,
   f. otoscope,
   g. transportation equipment (e.g., wheelchair, stretcher),
   h. equipment and supplies for pelvic examinations if female juveniles are housed in the facility, and

     i.   fetal heart monitor if pregnant juveniles are housed in the facility.

Basic equipment for on-site dental examinations includes, at a minimum:
- a. hand-washing facilities or appropriate alternate means of hand sanitization,
- b. dental examination chair,
- c. examination light,
- d. sterilizer,
- e. instruments,
- f. trash containers for biohazardous materials and sharps, and
- g. a dentist's stool.

Additionally, a dental operatory should have at least:
- a. an X-ray unit with developing capability,
- b. blood pressure monitoring equipment, and
- c. oxygen.

Optional Recommendations

It is good administrative practice to maintain inventory lists of all equipment, materials, and supplies purchased for health services.

Suitable medical and health care reference books, periodicals, audiotapes, videotapes, and online computer resources should be available to health staff. Publications should include current medical, mental health, dental, pharmacological, and nursing textbooks specific to the adolescent and developmental specialties, and a medical dictionary.

Y-D-04
important

DIAGNOSTIC SERVICES

Standard

On-site *diagnostic services* are registered, accredited, or otherwise meet applicable state and federal law.

Compliance Indicators

1. The responsible health authority maintains documentation that on-site diagnostic services (e.g., laboratory, radiology) are certified or licensed to provide that service.
2. When the facility provides on-site diagnostic services, there is a procedure manual for each service, including protocols for the calibration of testing devices to ensure accuracy.
3. Facilities with full-time health staff have multiple-test dipstick urinalysis, finger-stick blood glucose tests, peak flow meters (handheld or other), and in facilities housing female juveniles, pregnancy test kits.

4. All aspects of the standard are addressed by written policy and defined procedures.

Definition

Diagnostic services include biomedical or imaging services and results that are used to make clinical judgments. These diagnostic services may be provided by reference laboratories, hospital radiology and laboratory departments, public health agencies, or correctional facilities.

Discussion

An intent of this standard is that the facility provides the necessary diagnostic services for patient care. Specific resources for diagnostic studies and services to support the level of care provided to juveniles are important aspects of a comprehensive health care system.

Personnel working in radiology should regularly monitor levels of exposure through dosimeters.

Facilities offering on-site laboratory services should seek accreditation (or a waiver) by a CLIA-approved agency (Clinical Laboratory Improvement Amendments). The list of CLIA accrediting agencies can be obtained from the U.S. Department of Health and Human Services' Centers for Medicare and Medicaid Services.

Y-D-05
important

HOSPITAL AND SPECIALTY CARE

Standard

Arrangements are made to provide hospitalization and *specialty care* to patients in need of these services.

Compliance Indicators

1. For each community hospital or off-site specialty service used regularly for medical and mental health care, there is a *written agreement* that outlines the terms of the care to be provided.
2. The agreements require that the off-site facilities or health professionals provide a summary of the treatment given and any follow-up instructions; this information is to accompany the juvenile on return or be faxed immediately to facility health staff.
3. For on-site specialty services used regularly for medical and mental health care, there are appropriate licenses and certifications.
4. All aspects of the standard are addressed by written policy and defined procedures.

Definitions

Specialty care means specialist-provided health care (e.g., nephrology, surgery, dermatology, orthopedics).

Written agreement means a contract, letter of agreement, or memorandum of understanding between the facility and the hospital, clinic, or specialist for the care and treatment of patients.

Discussion

This standard intends that juveniles have access to necessary hospitalization and specialty services. Clinical need dictates the time required to receive the ordered service; in general, waiting times should not exceed average waiting times in community practice.

Specialty services provided on-site are in keeping with the legal requirements of the jurisdiction. Where certification, registration, licensure, or other authorization is to reflect that of equivalent community services, documentation of compliance by the facility is required.

To ensure continuity, the responsible health authority (RHA) anticipates and resolves problems in advance of the delivery of specialty care. The RHA addresses issues such as the commitment of the hospital, clinic, or specialist to see juveniles in its facility; general expectations regarding waiting times for appointments or admissions; specifics about what patient information is transferred between the RHA and the specialist; and the conditions and terms of payment. The RHA works with the facility authority regarding the procedures that transporting personnel follow while escorting patients for specialty care (see Y-E-10 Patient Escort). The RHA ensures that the patient is transferred to the hospital or clinic with a summary of the health record, and that a summary of the specialty care is received and filed in the patient's health record in the facility (see Y-H-01 Health Record Format and Contents). See also Y-A-01 Access to Care, Y-E-12 Continuity of Care During Incarceration, and Y-G-01 Chronic Disease Services regarding actual receipt of services.

SECTION E – JUVENILE CARE AND TREATMENT

Y-E-01
essential

INFORMATION ON HEALTH SERVICES

Standard

Information about the availability of, and access to, health care services is communicated orally and in writing to juveniles on their arrival at the facility, in a form and language they understand.

Compliance Indicators

1. A sign explaining how to access health services is posted in the intake / processing area.
2. Within 24 hours of their arrival, juveniles are given *written information* about:
   a. how to access emergency and routine medical, mental, and dental health services,
   b. the fee-for-service program, if one exists, and
   c. the grievance process for health-related complaints.
3. Special procedures ensure that juveniles who have difficulty communicating (e.g., foreign speaking, developmentally disabled, illiterate, mentally ill, deaf) understand how to access health services.
4. All aspects of the standard are addressed by written policy and defined procedures.

Definition

Written information may take the form of a facility handbook, a handout, or postings in juvenile housing areas.

Discussion

This standard intends that juveniles know about the availability of health care services and how to access them.

Information about health care services is basic to the provision of care in correctional settings and appropriate efforts are made to ensure that juveniles understand how they can access such services.

Optional Recommendations

Because the admission process may be stressful for incoming juveniles and they may not recall it clearly, it is good practice to provide new juveniles with a follow-up orientation to the health services program after they have settled in to the facility routine.

Arrangements should be made for an interpreter or an assistive device whenever effective communication is compromised due to speech, hearing, or language deficits. Selection of the interpreter or form of assistance should consider the patient's needs and abilities.

Y-E-02
essential

RECEIVING SCREENING

Standard

Receiving screening is performed on all juveniles on arrival at the intake facility to ensure that emergent and urgent health needs are met.

Compliance Indicators

1. Persons who are unconscious, semiconscious, bleeding, mentally unstable, or otherwise urgently in need of medical attention are:
    a. referred immediately for care and *medical clearance* into the facility, and
    b. if they are referred to a community hospital and then returned, their admission to the facility is predicated on written medical clearance from the hospital.
2. Immediate health needs are identified and addressed, and potentially infectious juveniles are isolated.
3. A *receiving screening* takes place for all juveniles *as soon as possible* by qualified health care professionals or health-trained child care staff.
4. When health-trained child care staff perform the receiving screening, they are to call health staff for disposition of the juvenile if problems are identified.
5. Reception personnel, using a form approved by the responsible health authority, conduct a basic receiving screening inquiry on:
    a. current and past illnesses, health conditions, and special health requirements (e.g., dietary needs);
    b. past serious infectious disease;
    c. recent communicable illness symptoms (e.g., chronic cough, coughing up blood, lethargy, weakness, weight loss, loss of appetite, fever, night sweats);
    d. past or current mental illness, including hospitalizations;
    e. history of or current suicidal ideation;
    f. dental problems;
    g. allergies;
    h. legal and illegal drug use (including type, amount, and time of last use);
    i. drug withdrawal symptoms;
    j. current or recent pregnancy; and
    k. other health problems as designated by the responsible physician.
6. Reception personnel record, on the receiving screening form, their screening observations of the juvenile's:
    a. appearance (e.g., sweating, tremors, anxious, disheveled),

    b.   behavior (e.g., disorderly, appropriate, insensible),

    c.   state of consciousness (e.g., alert, responsive, lethargic),

    d.   ease of movement (e.g., body deformities, gait),

    e.   breathing (e.g., persistent cough, hyperventilation), and

    f.   skin (including lesions, jaundice, rashes, infestations, bruises, scars, tattoos, and needle marks or other indications of drug abuse).

7.   The disposition of the juvenile (e.g., immediate referral to an appropriate health care service, placed in general population) is indicated on the receiving screening form.

8.   Receiving screening forms are dated and timed immediately on completion and include the signature and title of the person completing the form.

9.   Prescribed medications are reviewed and appropriately maintained according to the medication schedule the juvenile was following before admission.

10.   All aspects of the standard are addressed by written policy and defined procedures.

Definitions

Medical clearance is a clinical assessment of physical and mental status before an individual is admitted into the facility. Child care workers quickly inspect individuals to determine who may be too ill to wait for routine screening or to be admitted. Those identified to get immediate medical clearance are pulled from the group prior to admission. The medical clearance may come from on-site health staff or may require sending the individual to the local hospital emergency room. The medical clearance is to be documented in writing.

A *receiving screening* is conducted *as soon as possible*, it is promptly conducted without delay. Receiving screening personnel meet with each individual until all are processed. It is reasonable to expect that this will take time when there is a large group of juveniles. However, it is not acceptable to wait to start the screenings until child care staff complete the admission process. Individuals should not be released from the intake area until the receiving screening is completed.

Discussion

This standard is intended to fulfill four purposes: (1) to identify and meet any urgent health needs of those being admitted, (2) to identify and meet any known or easily identifiable health needs that require medical intervention prior to the health assessment (see Y-E-04 Health Assessment), (3) to identify and isolate juveniles who appear potentially contagious, and (4) to obtain a medical clearance when necessary.

At times facilities receive newly arriving juveniles in large groups, making it impossible to screen each juvenile immediately. Screening can be viewed as consisting of two stages: medical clearance and receiving screening.

Receiving screening is a process of structured inquiry and observation designed to prevent newly arrived juveniles who pose a threat to their own or others' health or safety from being admitted to the facility's general population. It is intended to identify potential emergency situations among new arrivals, and to ensure that patients with known illnesses and currently on medications are identified for further assessment and continued treatment. It is conducted using a form and language fully understood by the juvenile, who may not speak English or may have a physical (e.g., speech, hearing, sight) or mental disability.

For juveniles identified as having pulmonary tuberculosis, isolation from the general juvenile population and immediate treatment for the disease are required.

Screeners are to make adequate efforts to explore the potential for suicide. Both reviewing with a juvenile any history of suicidal behavior and visually observing the juvenile's behavior (delusions, hallucinations, communication difficulties, speech and posture, impaired level of consciousness, disorganization, memory defects, depression, or evidence of self-mutilation) are done. The screeners also look for symptoms of withdrawal from alcohol and other drugs and the potential that they might develop later. These approaches, coupled with training in aspects of mental health and chemical dependency, enable staff to intervene early to treat withdrawal and to prevent most suicides (see Y-G-05 Suicide Prevention Program and Y-G-06 Intoxication and Withdrawal).

Particular attention is to be paid to signs of trauma. Staff members have a responsibility to report suspected abuse of juveniles to the appropriate authorities. Juveniles arriving with signs of recent trauma are referred immediately for medical observation and treatment.

Although it is recommended that health professionals conduct the initial screening, this standard allows receiving screening to be conducted by health-trained child care workers. The training these workers are given depends on the role they are expected to play in the receiving screening process. At a minimum, they receive instruction on how to take a medical history, how to make the required observations, how to determine the appropriate disposition of a juvenile based on responses to questions and observations, and how to document their findings on the receiving screening form. Because newly arrived juveniles may need urgent medical assistance, child care workers in the reception area are to have current training in first aid and CPR.

Optional Recommendations

Juveniles with mental disorders are often unable to give complete or accurate information in response to health status inquiries. Therefore, mental health staff should be involved in training the staff who do the intake screening.

The facility should follow a tuberculosis control plan consistent with current published guidelines from the Centers for Disease Control and Prevention.

It is recommended that selected early detection and treatment services be initiated for sexually transmitted infections (STIs; e.g., chlamydia, gonorrhea, HIV, syphilis). Current STI screening technology allows for the detection of some infections within a few hours of admission, which may lead to prompt treatment before juveniles infect others in the facility or in the community. The intent of this recommendation is to offer solutions to problems that may develop without early intervention. For example, infected and untreated juveniles of childbearing age, when released into the community, may develop costly and painful STI complications, including adverse outcomes of pregnancy.

Performance Measures

1. When a health problem is identified after admission that should have been identified during the receiving screening but was not, a continuing quality improvement (CQI) analysis of the root cause is initiated.
2. When a health problem identified during receiving screening is not communicated to appropriate staff, a CQI analysis of the root cause is initiated.
3. Where indicated, appropriate action is taken to mitigate any negative outcome for the juvenile involved.

Performance Measure Expectations

The expectation is that the performance measures are met 100% of the time.

"CQI analysis" refers to methods of studying a problem or process that identifies factors that may be contributing to the difficulty being studied. "Root cause(s)" refers to the basic factor(s) that are the reason for the difficulty. The RHA decides what methods of study and documentation are to be used in internal reviews to assess compliance with these measures. All such studies and tracking methods are incorporated into the facility's CQI program.

Both measures for the receiving screening process look at how well health problems are identified at reception and communicated to appropriate health staff, with the outcome that juveniles receive the health care required. Evaluation of facility performance can be accomplished by, for example, keeping a log in which a practitioner records the details of when he or she discovers a health problem that should have been identified during the receiving screening (measure #1) or discovers a lack of communication about a health condition (measure #2). Such a log will enable designated staff to follow up and identify where the process went wrong. This method of identifying problems is ongoing and directly linked to caregiver interactions with the patient.

Record reviews also can be structured to trace current health problems back to when they were first identified, a method that would also highlight any gaps in the continuum from receiving screening to treatment.

For further information, see Appendix B – Compliance Indicators and Performance Measures.

Y-E-03
essential

TRANSFER SCREENING

Standard

A transfer screening is performed on all *intrasystem transfers*.

Compliance Indicators

1. Qualified health care professionals or health care liaisons review each incoming juvenile's health record or summary within 12 hours of arrival:
   a. continuity of care is initiated,
   b. missing initial assessments (health, mental health, dental) are identified and any required assessments are scheduled, and
   c. records from the sending facility are filed in the current health record.
2. The receiving screening for transfers takes place upon the juvenile's arrival at the facility.
   a. Where the health record or a health information transfer summary comes with the juvenile and is immediately available to the screening staff, a face-to-face transfer screening encounter focuses on observation of appearance and behavior, and problems the juvenile recounts that occurred during the transfer process.
   b. Where the health record or health information transfer summary is not available to the screening staff, a face-to-face transfer screening encounter, at a minimum, includes:
      i. identification of acute and chronic health conditions,
      ii. evaluation of suicidal risk,
      iii. review of any allergies,
      iv. observation of appearance and behavior, and
      v. problems the juvenile recounts that occurred during the transfer process.
3. Documentation of the transfer screening is dated and timed immediately upon completion and includes the signature and title of the person completing the process.
4. All aspects of the standard are addressed by written policy and defined procedures.

Definition

Intrasystem transfers include juveniles being transferred from one facility to another within the same correctional authority's system.

Discussion

This standard is intended to ensure that juveniles continue to receive appropriate health services for health needs already identified and that unnecessary repetitive tests are avoided when juveniles are transferred between separate facilities that are part of the same correctional system.

Because of the unpredictability of juveniles in general, the transfer screening includes a face-to-face evaluation by the trained facility or health staff.

Optional Recommendation

Documentation of the transfer screening process is best recorded on a standardized form or in a uniform format.

Y-E-04
essential

HEALTH ASSESSMENT

Standard

Juveniles receive initial and periodic *health assessments*.

Compliance Indicators

1. As soon as possible, but no later than 7 calendar days after admission to the facility, an initial health assessment is completed on each juvenile.
2. The initial health assessment includes, but is not limited to:
   a. review of the receiving screening results;
   b. collection of additional data to complete the medical, dental, and mental health histories;
   c. review of immunization history and update of schedules as needed;
   d. recording of vital signs (i.e., height, weight, pulse, blood pressure, and temperature);
   e. physical examination (including breast, rectal, and genitourinary exams as indicated by gender, age, and risk factors);
   f. gynecological assessment of females, when clinically indicated;
   g. laboratory and/or diagnostic tests for communicable diseases, including sexually transmitted infections as determined by the responsible physician with recommendations from the local public health department; and
   h. initiation of therapy when appropriate.

3. The responsible physician determines the frequency and content of periodic health assessments on the basis of protocols promulgated by nationally recognized professional organizations.
4. A health history, which includes information on the juvenile's participation in risky behavior, including sexual activity, is collected by qualified health care professionals.
5. The hands-on portion of the health assessment is performed by a physician, physician assistant, nurse practitioner, or other practitioner as permitted by law. When significant findings are present, the responsible physician documents his or her review of health assessments done by a physician assistant, nurse practitioner, or other practitioner.
6. The hands-on portion of the health assessment may be performed by a registered nurse when:
    a. the nurse completes appropriate training, approved or provided by the responsible physician, and
    b. the responsible physician documents his or her review of all health assessments.
7. The responsible health authority approves the health assessment form.
8. All aspects of the standard are addressed by written policy and defined procedures.

Definitions

The *health assessment* is the process whereby an individual's health status is evaluated, including questioning the patient about symptoms. The extent of the health assessment is defined by the responsible physician but should include at least the steps noted in this standard.

A *physical examination* is an objective, hands-on evaluation of an individual. It involves the inspection, palpation, auscultation, and percussion of a patient's body to determine the presence or absence of physical signs of disease.

Discussion

This standard intends that health care professionals assess and plan for meeting the health needs of the individual.

Juveniles are appropriately evaluated to prevent chronic disorders, communicable disease, and mental illness from going undetected in the facility. The health assessment also provides an excellent opportunity to initiate preventive medicine practices and provide health education. Juveniles are advised of the need for a health assessment in a manner that encourages participation.

The evaluation includes a medical history, physical examination, and diagnostic testing. Testing for communicable disease such as tuberculosis or sexually transmitted infections occurs for all juveniles unless the responsible physician and local public health authority determine this is not necessary.

Clusters of medical signs or symptoms in a patient may indicate a need for a mental health assessment.

Certain elements of the health assessment are repeated at an appropriate frequency as determined by the responsible physician in consideration of the age, gender, and health need, consistent with the recommendations of professional organizations. Such organizations include the American Academy of Family Physicians, the American Academy of Pediatrics, the American Cancer Society, the American College of Obstetricians and Gynecologists, and the American Medical Association.

Health assessments are not required for all juveniles readmitted to the facility when the last health assessment was performed within 12 months and when the juvenile's new receiving screening shows no change in health status. The juvenile is seen by the physician, who assesses the need for further health evaluation. When appropriate, histories, physical examinations, and tests are updated.

Optional Recommendation

When various parts of the assessment are done by different health staff, the responsible physician ensures that the evaluations are integrated.

Performance Measures

1. Health assessments are completed within 7 days of the juvenile's arrival at the facility.
2. When a health problem is identified after the initial health assessment that should have been identified during the initial assessment but was not, a continuous quality improvement (CQI) analysis of the root cause is initiated.
3. Where indicated, appropriate action is taken to mitigate any negative outcome for the juvenile involved.

Performance Measure Expectations

The expectation is that the performance measures are met 100% of the time.

"CQI analysis" refers to methods of studying a problem or process that identifies various factors involved that may be contributing to the difficulty being studied. "Root cause(s)" refers to the basic factor(s) that are the reason for the difficulty studied. The RHA decides what methods of study and documentation are to be used in the internal reviews to assess compliance with these measures. All such studies and tracking methods are incorporated into the facility's CQI program.

Measure #1 can be assessed, for example, by keeping lists or logs that include dates of admission and the health assessment.

Measure #2 requires the practitioner to check the juvenile's initial health assessment each time a new health problem is identified that, with good medical practice, should have been picked up during the initial health assessment. Evaluation of how well the facility is doing can be accomplished by keeping a log that requires the current treating practitioner to record particulars that enable designated staff to follow up and identify where the process went wrong. This method of identifying problems is ongoing and directly linked to caregiver interactions with the patient.

Record reviews can also be structured to trace current health problems back to when they were first identified, a method that would also highlight any gaps in the initial health assessment process.

Y-E-05
essential

MENTAL HEALTH SCREENING AND EVALUATION

Standard

All juveniles receive mental health screening; juveniles with positive screens receive a mental health evaluation.

Compliance Indicators

1. Within 14 days of admission to the correctional system, qualified mental health professionals or *mental health staff* conduct initial mental health screening.
2. The initial mental health screening includes a structured interview with inquiries into:
   a. a history of:
      i. psychiatric hospitalization and outpatient treatment,
      ii. suicidal behavior,
      iii. *violent behavior,*
      iv. victimization, including physical and sexual abuse,
      v. special education placement,
      vi. cerebral trauma or seizures,
      vii. sex offenses, and
      viii. exposure to traumatic life events and losses;
   b. the current status of:
      i. psychotropic medications,
      ii. suicidal ideation,
      iii. drug or alcohol use, and
      iv. orientation to person, place, and time;
   c. emotional response to incarceration; and

       d.   a screening for *intellectual functioning* (i.e., mental retardation, developmental disability, learning disability).

3.   The patient's health record contains results of the initial screening.

4.   Juveniles who screen positive for mental health problems are referred to *qualified mental health professionals* for further evaluation.

5.   The health record contains results of the evaluation with documentation of referral or initiation of treatment when indicated.

6.   Patients who require acute mental health services beyond those available on site are transferred to an appropriate facility.

7.   There is a written policy and defined procedures addressing the postadmission mental health screening and evaluation process.

Definitions

Mental health staff include qualified health care professionals who have received instruction and supervision in identifying and interacting with individuals in need of mental health services.

Qualified mental health professionals include psychiatrists, psychologists, psychiatric social workers, psychiatric nurses, and others who by virtue of their education, credentials, and experience are permitted by law to evaluate and care for the mental health needs of patients.

Violent behavior is defined as *expressive violence* initiated as a result of an interpersonal altercation where the goal is to injure the other person, or as *instrumental violence* where the goal is to get something from the person (usually the result of criminal intent). An understanding of the history of either form of violence and the circumstances leading to the specific behavior is helpful in assessing the patient's potential for further violent behavior.

Screening for *intellectual functioning* includes inquiry into history of developmental and educational difficulties and, when indicated, referral for application of standardized psychological intelligence tools as appropriate.

Discussion

This standard intends to ensure that the juvenile's serious mental health needs, including those related to developmental disability and/or addictions, are identified.

The postadmission mental health screening is completed in addition to the mental health portion of the receiving screening (see Y-E-02 Receiving Screening). Mentally ill and developmentally disabled juveniles are to be identified soon after admission to prevent deterioration in their level of functioning and to receive necessary treatment in a timely fashion (see Y-G-04 Basic Mental Health Services).

When appropriate, additional investigation is carried out regarding the abuse of alcohol and/or drugs, including the type of substances abused, modes of use, amounts used, frequency of use, and date or time of last use; current or previous treatment for alcohol or drug abuse, if any, and when and where; whether the juvenile is taking medication for an alcohol or drug abuse problem; and current or past illnesses and health problems related to substance abuse, such as hepatitis, seizures, traumatic injuries, infections, and liver diseases.

Optional Recommendation

It is recommended that juveniles identified as possibly retarded on group tests of intelligence or brief intelligence screening instruments be further evaluated by a comprehensive, individually administered instrument such as the Wechsler Intelligence Scale for Children (WISC).

Y-E-06
essential

ORAL CARE

Standard

Oral care under the direction and supervision of a dentist licensed in the state is provided to each juvenile. Care is timely and includes immediate access for urgent or painful conditions. There is a system of established priorities for care when, in the dentist's judgment, the juvenile's health would otherwise be adversely affected.

Compliance Indicators

1. *Oral screening* by the dentist or qualified health care professionals trained by the dentist is performed within 7 days of admission.
2. Instruction in oral hygiene and preventive oral education are given within 14 days of admission.
3. An *oral examination* is performed by a dentist within 60 days of admission.
4. *Oral treatment*, not limited to extractions, is provided according to a treatment plan based on a system of established priorities for care when, in the dentist's judgment, the juvenile's health would otherwise be adversely affected.
5. Radiographs are appropriately used in the development of the treatment plan.
6. Consultation through referral to oral health care specialists is available as needed.
7. Each juvenile has access to the preventive benefits of fluorides in a form determined by the dentist to be appropriate for the needs of the individual.
8. Where oral care is provided on site, contemporary *infection control* procedures are followed.
9. Extractions are performed in a manner consistent with community standards of care and adhering to the American Dental Association's clinical guidelines.

10. All aspects of the standard are addressed by written policy and defined procedures.

Definitions

Oral care includes instruction in oral hygiene, examination, and treatment of dental problems. Instruction in oral hygiene minimally includes information on plaque control and the proper brushing of teeth.

Oral screening includes visual observation of the teeth and gums, and notation of any obvious or gross abnormalities requiring immediate referral to a dentist.

Oral examination by a dentist includes taking or reviewing the patient's oral history, an extraoral head and neck examination, charting of teeth, and examination of the hard and soft tissue of the oral cavity with a mouth mirror, explorer, and adequate illumination.

Oral treatment includes the full range of services that in the supervising dentist's judgment are necessary for proper mastication and maintaining the juvenile's health status.

Infection control practices are defined by the American Dental Association and the Centers for Disease Control and Prevention as including sterilizing instruments, disinfecting equipment, and properly disposing of hazardous waste.

Discussion

This standard intends that juveniles' serious dental needs are met.

As in medical or mental health care, dental care is based on patient need. Oral care is an important component of an individual's overall health care. Poor oral health has been linked to numerous systemic diseases.

Oral screening can be performed as part of the intake process. Where nondental qualified health care professionals do the initial oral screening, there is documentation of their training by a dentist. Such training consists of more than completion of self-study programs.

Oral hygiene instruction and preventive oral education are given by dentists, dental hygienists, or dentally trained personnel, and consist of measures to assist the patient in caring for his or her own oral health.

Dental examinations and treatment are performed only by licensed dental personnel. In the case of a readmitted juvenile who has received an oral examination in the correctional system within the past year, a new exam is not required except as determined by the supervising dentist.

Optional Recommendations

The dental treatment plan should identify existing dental needs, denote proposed dental treatment, and include a periodontal evaluation.

Patient noncompliance with good oral hygiene practices (e.g., plaque control) should not be used as a basis to deny needed oral care. Assistance should be provided for juveniles who, because of mental, physical, or other disabilities, are unable to perform daily oral hygiene techniques.

Y-E-07
essential

NONEMERGENCY HEALTH CARE REQUESTS AND SERVICES

Standard

All juveniles have the opportunity *daily* to request health care. Their *requests* are documented and reviewed for immediacy of need and the intervention required. *Sick call* and *clinicians' clinics* are conducted on a timely basis and in a *clinical setting* by qualified health care professionals.

Compliance Indicators

1. Oral or written requests for health care are received daily by qualified health care professionals and *triaged* within 24 hours. Based on physician-approved protocols, qualified health care professionals schedule juveniles, when indicated, for sick call or the next available clinician's clinic. When qualified health care professionals are not on duty within a 24-hour period, health-trained child care staff, using facility protocols established by the legal and health authorities, review and respond to juveniles' health care requests (see Y-C-08 Health Care Liaison).
2. During sick call, qualified health care professionals make timely assessments in a clinical setting. Based on physician-approved protocols, qualified health care professionals provide treatment according to clinical priorities or, when indicated, schedule patients for the next available clinician's clinic.
3. All juveniles, regardless of housing assignment, have access to regularly scheduled sick call.
4. The frequency and duration of sick call are sufficient to meet the health needs of the juvenile population, generally three times a week given the time frames of indicator #1.
5. All aspects of the standard are addressed by written policy and defined procedures.

Definitions

Daily means 7 days a week including holidays.

Request for health care refers to oral or written petitions for medical, dental, or mental health services. These requests are to be documented.

Sick call is the evaluation and treatment of an ambulatory patient in a clinical setting, either on or off site, by a qualified health care professional.

Clinician's clinic is sick call held by physicians, nurse practitioners, physician assistants, dentists, or mental health clinicians.

Clinical setting refers to an examination or treatment room appropriately supplied and equipped to address the patient's health care needs (see Y-D-03 Clinic Space, Equipment, and Supplies).

Triage is the sorting and classifying of juveniles' health requests to determine priority of need and the proper place for health care to be rendered.

Discussion

This standard intends that juveniles' routine health care needs are met.

The RHA has a system that enables all juveniles to request health services daily. There are many systems that satisfy this standard. Juveniles can access the health care system by walking into a clinic and making an appointment, writing their request on slips that are dropped into a locked box (these are picked up by health staff who go to all housing areas), telephoning a nurse in the clinic, or using sign-up sheets in the dining hall or housing area. In all cases, care should be taken to protect the confidentiality of juveniles' health problems.

Nonemergency requests are to be reviewed within 24 hours and the juvenile seen by a qualified health care professional at sick call within the next 24 hours (72 hours on weekends). A disposition is made and noted on the sick-call slip, log or appointment book (e.g., scheduled for next sick call, dental appointment made, referred to psychologist). Not every sick-call request requires a sick-call appointment; however, when a request describes a clinical symptom, a face-to-face encounter between the juvenile and a health professional is required. This applies to mental health and dental symptoms, as well.

The frequency and duration of sick call may vary according to facility size. Correctional facilities with a high proportion of segregated juveniles or special needs patients may require more frequent sick calls or extended hours to accommodate all requests and needs.

When indicated, referral to the clinician's clinic is made for the juvenile to see a physician or midlevel practitioner. In general, when a juvenile reports to sick call more than two times with the same complaint and has not seen a physician, he or she receives an appointment to do so.

Optional Recommendations

Because better disposition decisions are likely to result, qualified health care professionals with the most experience should triage juvenile health care requests. Indicators such as a high number of grievances or a high number of hospital emergency room visits may point to the need for increased physician time.

Y-E-08
essential

EMERGENCY SERVICES

Standard

The facility provides 24-hour *emergency* medical, mental health, and dental services.

Compliance Indicators

1. A written plan includes arrangements for the following, which are carried out when necessary:
   a. emergency transport of the patient from the facility,
   b. use of an emergency medical vehicle,
   c. use of one or more designated hospital emergency departments or other appropriate facilities,
   d. emergency on-call physician, mental health, and dental services when the emergency health care facility is not nearby,
   e. security procedures for the immediate transfer of patients for emergency medical care, and
   f. notification to the person legally responsible for the facility.
2. Emergency drugs, supplies, and medical equipment are regularly maintained.
3. All aspects of the standard are addressed by written policy and defined procedures.

Definitions

Emergency medical, mental health, and dental health care is care for an acute illness or an unexpected health need that cannot be deferred until the next scheduled sick call or clinic.

Automated external defibrillators (AEDs) are electronic devices that interpret cardiac rhythms and, if necessary, deliver an electrical shock to the patient.

Discussion

This standard intends that sufficient emergency health planning occurs and is put into effect when necessary. Planning ahead for emergencies can help minimize bad outcomes. Policy and procedures address, for example, which on-call staff need to be notified, arranging for an ambulance, and alerting the community emergency room.

All members of the health and child care staff on all shifts who have direct contact with the juveniles should be familiar with the procedures for obtaining emergency medical care and responding to emergencies. It is not necessary for nonhealth staff to wait for health staff to arrive before activating emergency response procedures or initiating emergency intervention. Training is given so that the first person on the scene intervenes until facility health staff or community emergency responders arrive. The names, addresses, and telephone numbers of people to be notified and/or services (such as ambulance and hospital) to be used should be readily accessible to all personnel.

Unless the clinicians live on the facility grounds, the response to a true medical emergency includes activation of the community emergency medical system.

The choice of basic emergency equipment depends on the size of the facility, its distance from the nearest emergency department, and the level of staff training.

Optional Recommendations

The availability of emergency services should be considered when assigning juveniles with known medical conditions to facilities in remote areas. Facilities from which the trip to an emergency room would take longer than 15 minutes via ambulance should not house juveniles with significant health problems.

Modern AEDs are designed to be applied by medical and nonmedical personnel with little or no training. They are increasingly being used in the community and should be considered in all correctional settings. Correctional administrators and medical directors considering the use of AEDs should identify when the devices are to be used, who should be trained in their use, and where they should be kept. The use of AEDs should be approved, planned, and implemented under the direction of the responsible physician in collaboration with the facility authority.

Performance Measures

1. When medical emergencies occur, the appropriate emergency response is initiated.
2. There is evidence of full compliance with the schedules for maintenance of emergency supplies, drugs, and medical equipment as outlined in the emergency response plan.

Performance Measure Expectations

The expectation is that the performance measures are met 100% of the time.

The RHA decides what methods of study and documentation are to be used in internal reviews to assess compliance with these measures. All such studies and tracking methods are incorporated into the facility's continuous quality improvement program.

Measure #1 requires keeping aggregate data incorporating information from the critiques and debriefings that are already required in order to complete the drill process.

Measure #2 can be documented using any method the facility chooses to confirm that the required inspections or maintenance of equipment is completed.

Y-E-09
essential

SEGREGATED JUVENILES

Standard

When a juvenile is *segregated*, health staff monitor his or her health.

Compliance Indicators

1. Upon notification that a juvenile is placed in segregation:
    a. a qualified health care professional reviews the juvenile's health record to determine whether existing medical, dental, or mental health needs contraindicate the placement or require accommodation. Such review is documented in the health record.
    b. When health staff are not on duty, the health staff member on call is notified.
2. When on duty, health professionals monitor segregated juveniles daily by performing *health checks*.
    a. The daily health monitoring may be done by either medical or mental health professionals.
    b. Mental health staff see juveniles on their active case load at least weekly.
    c. Child care workers or program staff monitor juveniles in segregation at least every 15 minutes.
    d. On days when health staff are not on site, health-trained child care workers or program staff alert health staff on call if a health problem is noted.
3. In the rare instance that a segregated juvenile's out-of-control behavior lasts 24 hours, qualified health care professionals evaluate the juvenile directly and:
    a. approve continued isolation, or
    b. generate a written plan for urgent mental health assessment by a qualified mental health professional and/or the use of alternatives to segregation (e.g., return to living units under supervision, use of medications, transfer to a mental health facility).

4. Documentation of segregation rounds is made on individual logs or room cards, or in the juvenile's health record, and includes:
   a. the date and time of the contact, and
   b. the signature or initials of the health staff member making the rounds.
5. Any significant health findings are documented in the juvenile's health record.
6. A monthly report on the use of segregation is given to the responsible health authority (RHA) and facility administrator. This report should include information about the number of juveniles in segregation during the month, the number of days spent in segregation, and the health status of segregated juveniles.
7. All aspects of the standard are addressed by written policy and defined procedures.

Definitions

Health checks required by the standard are face-to-face encounters with the segregated juvenile to ascertain medical and mental health status and provide an opportunity for requests for health care. When problems are noted, appropriate clinical interventions are initiated that may include the discontinuation of segregation for health reasons.

Segregated juveniles are those isolated from the general population and who receive services and activities apart from other juveniles. Facilities may refer to juveniles housed in such conditions as being in administrative segregation, protective custody, or disciplinary segregation. For the purposes of this standard, the living and confinement conditions define the segregated status, not the reason a juvenile was placed in segregation.

This standard does not apply to medical isolation as ordered by a physician, or mental health "time out" as directed in an individual treatment plan.

Degree of disease control refers to how well the disease or illness is being treated so that the symptoms do not interfere with daily living and related complications do not develop. The following common chronic illnesses are to be monitored: asthma, diabetes, epilepsy, high blood cholesterol, high blood pressure, and HIV. (See Y-G-01 Chronic Disease Services).

Discussion

The intent of this standard is to ensure that juveniles placed in segregation maintain their medical and mental health while physically and socially isolated from the remainder of the juvenile population.

Checks by health staff ensure that each segregated juvenile has the opportunity to request care for medical, dental, and mental health problems. In addition, by visiting with the juvenile during these checks, health staff are able to ascertain the juvenile's general medical and mental health status.

This standard reflects a number of findings and assumptions:

Segregation is a behavioral control measure (thus subject to administrative responsibility) that may pose medical danger (thus subject to medical responsibility). This danger increases as segregation is prolonged.

The decision to place a juvenile in segregation should be left to the discretion of trained program staff, but this action should precipitate a series of monitoring actions by health personnel to protect the segregated juvenile from harm. The longer a juvenile remains in segregation, the greater the role of the health staff should be in the decision-making process. In the beginning, health staff involvement should be confined to monitoring the juvenile's psychological state, but as the segregation period lengthens, health personnel should take appropriate action with regard to the juvenile's health status.

Prolonged segregation is defined by scientific research, community standards, regulations, statutes, and case law. In cases where litigation has determined the upper limit for segregating juveniles, judges have imposed ranges of 2 to 5 hours. Successful experiences of juvenile detention and confinement programs that have strict limits on isolation indicate that the vast majority of segregation events can be limited to minutes or hours, and the use of segregation for a day or more is unnecessary in all but a few cases.

When a segregated juvenile requests health care, arrangements are made for triage, examination, and treatment in an appropriate clinical setting. The segregation rounds are required in addition to whatever mechanism is in place to request health services daily (see Y-E-07 Nonemergency Health Care Requests and Services).

Special attention is given to vulnerable populations such as the mentally ill. Care is taken when reviewing health records of juveniles with serious mental health illnesses to assess the risk of exacerbation of the mental illness. Health staff reviewing the record notify mental health staff when the juvenile is currently under the care of mental health services.

Due to the possibility of injury and depression during isolation, the evaluations by health staff include notation of bruises or other trauma markings, comments regarding the juvenile's attitude and outlook (particularly as they might relate to suicidal ideation), and any health complaints.

Necessary clinical encounters take place in an appropriate clinical setting (not room-side) and are noted in each patient's health record.

Documentation of segregation rounds can be done on individual logs or room cards that, when filled, are filed in the juvenile's health record.

Optional Recommendations

In recognition of the deleterious effects of prolonged segregation on juveniles, it is recommended that health staff be involved in the development and/or review of segregation policies and procedures so that appropriate accommodations for health conditions can be addressed.

Segregation policies should state that this intervention is to be reserved for incidents in which the juvenile's behavior has escalated beyond the staff's ability to control the juvenile by counseling or disciplinary measures and presents a risk of injury to the juvenile or others.

If special (nonresidential) rooms are used for segregation, they should be as well-illuminated as regular unit rooms and have easy access to appropriate toilet facilities.

Although administrators and health personnel may wish to see segregation as an exclusive administrative measure, judges consistently have declared it a medical procedure on the basis of its medical dangers. Health staff, therefore, are strongly encouraged to learn about the risks of segregation and appropriate safeguards against its misuse. It is the responsibility of health care personnel to inform the facility administrator about any misuse of segregation.

Performance Measures

1. Daily monitoring by health staff occurs for segregated juvenile.
2. For segregated juveniles with chronic disease(s), including mental health conditions, the *degree of disease control* does not worsen. (See the Performance Measure Expectations for examples.) The RHA may choose to study one or more diseases to review, and does not have to study all of the diseases at any one time.

Performance Measure Expectations

The expectation is that the performance measures are met 100% of the time.

The RHA decides what methods of study and documentation are to be used in their internal reviews to assess their compliance with these measures. All such studies and tracking methods are incorporated into the facility's CQI program.

Measure #1 can be documented in many ways provided that information reflects actual daily practice for all segregated juvenile. This enables periodic and aggregate data to be compiled and reviewed.

Measure #2 requires special individualized health status evaluation and tracking and a reporting mechanism that includes both individual and aggregate data presentation.

Y-E-10
important

PATIENT ESCORT

Standard

Patients are transported safely and in a timely manner for medical, mental health, and dental clinic appointments both inside and outside the facility.

Compliance Indicators

1. When a patient is escorted, health staff alert transporting child care staff to accommodations needed during the transport process, including instructions for administration of necessary medications.
2. Patient confidentiality is maintained during transport.
3. All aspects of the standard are addressed by written policy and defined procedures.

Discussion

An intent of this standard is that the facility provides sufficient escorting staff so that patients can meet scheduled health care appointments. The principle of access to care rests on the ability of juveniles to request and receive health services in a timely fashion. When required for security purposes, child care worker administration ensures that personnel are available to escort patients from housing to clinic areas for their scheduled appointments.

When warranted (e.g., for segregated juveniles), qualified health care professionals may see patients in the housing unit provided that the health encounter is conducted in a clinical setting (see Y-E-07 Nonemergency Health Care Requests and Services).

When patients visit health professionals outside the facility, child care worker and health staff ensure that the transports are conducted on a timely basis. All patient transports, regardless of the reason, occur in a manner that maintains the confidentiality of health information and ensures adequate care consistent with the patient's health needs (see Y-A-09 Privacy of Care and Y-H-02 Confidentiality of Health Records and Information). If applicable, a sufficient supply of medication is made available to the patient during transport.

Optional Recommendations

Health staff should record missed appointments, including rescheduling information, and a monthly report of unkept scheduled clinic appointments should be given to the responsible health authority. The responsible health authority should monitor the cause(s) of all scheduled but unmet clinic appointments (e.g., conflict in work or school, resolution of health complaint, court appearances, lack of facility personnel for transport).

Y-E-11
important

NURSING ASSESSMENT PROTOCOLS

Standard

Nursing assessment protocols are appropriate to the level of skill and preparation of the nursing personnel who will carry them out, and comply with the relevant state practice acts. *Standing orders* may be used only for preventive medicine practices.

Compliance Indicators

1. Protocols are developed and reviewed annually by the nursing administrator and responsible physician.
2. Documentation of nurses' training in protocol use exists. This includes:
   a. evidence that all new nursing staff are trained,
   b. demonstration of knowledge and skills,
   c. evidence of annual review of skills, and
   d. evidence of retraining when protocols are introduced or revised.
3. Nursing assessment protocols do not include the use of prescription medications except for those covering emergency, life-threatening situations (e.g., nitroglycerin, epinephrine). Emergency administration of these medications requires a subsequent clinician's order.
4. All aspects of the standard are addressed by written policy and defined procedures.

Definitions

Nursing assessment protocols are written instructions or guidelines that specify the steps to be taken in evaluating a patient's health status and providing interventions. Such protocols may include acceptable first-aid procedures for the identification and care of ailments that ordinarily would be treated by an individual with over-the-counter medication or through self-care. They also may address more serious symptoms such as chest pain, shortness of breath, and intoxication. They specify a sequence of steps to be taken to evaluate and stabilize the patient until a clinician is contacted and orders are received for further care.

Standing orders are written orders that specify the same course of treatment for each patient suspected of having a given condition, and that specify the use and amount of prescription drugs.

Discussion

This standard intends to ensure that nurses who provide clinical services are trained and do so under specified guidelines. Nursing assessment protocols can be helpful in the clinical management of patients. The protocols have a signed declaration indicating that they have been reviewed and approved by the nursing administrator and responsible physician. When protocols are changed, they are to be individually dated and signed by the nursing administrator and the responsible physician.

Treatment protocols or algorithms used by clinicians such as physicians, physician assistants, nurse practitioners, or psychologists are not included in this standard. Such treatment protocols comply with regulations set forth by state boards and national practice professional organizations, and are approved by the responsible physician.

Treatment with prescription medication is initiated only on the written or oral order of a licensed clinician. Standing orders are not used except for preventive medicine practices (e.g., immunizations) that are in keeping with current community practice.

Y-E-12
essential

CONTINUITY OF CARE DURING INCARCERATION

Standard

Juveniles receive treatment and diagnostic tests ordered by clinicians.

Compliance Indicators

1. When diagnostic tests and specialty consultations are ordered:
   a. they are completed in a timely manner,
   b. the ordering clinician's review of results is documented in the record, and
   c. the clinician reviews the findings with the patient in a timely manner.
2. When a juvenile returns from an emergency room (ER) visit, the physician sees the patient, reviews the discharge orders, and issues follow-up orders as clinically indicated. If the physician is not on site, designated health staff contact the physician on-call to review ER findings and obtain orders as appropriate.
3. When a juvenile returns from hospitalization, the physician sees the patient, reviews the discharge orders, and issues follow-up orders as clinically indicated. If the physician is not on site, designated staff immediately review the hospital's discharge instructions and contact the facility physician for orders as needed.
4. Clinicians use diagnostic and treatment results to modify treatment plans as appropriate.

5. If changes in treatment are indicated, the changes are implemented or clinical justification for an alternative course is noted.

6. Individual treatment plans are used to guide treatment for episodes of illness. The format for the planning may vary, but should include, at a minimum:

    a. the frequency of follow-up for medical evaluation and adjustment of treatment modality,

    b. the type and frequency of diagnostic testing and therapeutic regimens, and

    c. when appropriate, instructions about diet, exercise, adaptation to the correctional environment, and medication.

7. *Physician clinical chart reviews* are of sufficient number and frequency to ensure that clinically appropriate care is ordered and implemented by on-site health staff.

8. All aspects of the standard are addressed by written policy and defined procedures.

Discussion

The intent of this standard is to ensure that patients receive health services in keeping with current community standards as ordered by clinicians.

Continuity of care is a broad concept that encompasses many issues also addressed elsewhere in the Standards. (See Y-D-02 Medication Services, Y-E-02 Receiving Screening, Y-E-03 Transfer Screening, Y-E-04 Health Assessment, Y-E-05 Mental Health Screening and Evaluation, Y-E-06 Oral Care, Y-E-13 Discharge Planning, Y-G-01 Chronic Disease Services, and Y-G-02 Patients With Special Health Needs.) This standard, however, focuses directly on the treating clinician's professional responsibilities to ensure continuity of care from admission to discharge and is of concern in all areas of health care—medical, mental health, and dental.

In a proactive health services program, clinician visits are automatically scheduled following diagnostic testing, specialty consultation, ER visits, and hospitalization. Qualified health care professionals review the medical orders and instructions when a juvenile returns from an off-site health facility. This review ensures continuity of care, and the visits also serve as a safety net to ensure that any treatment recommendations are reviewed, followed, or revised as appropriate.

Episodes of acute illness are resolved more quickly and negative health consequences avoided when the treatment is planned, documented, and monitored. The planning may be recorded on specific forms or in the progress notes, with outcomes recorded until the health issue is resolved.

Physician clinical chart review is an evaluation by a physician of the timeliness and appropriateness of the clinical care provided to patients. The number and frequency of chart reviews are expected to increase if significant problems are identified.

Y-E-13
important

DISCHARGE PLANNING

Standard

Discharge planning is provided for juveniles with serious health needs whose release is imminent.

Compliance Indicators

1. For planned discharges, health staff:
    a. coordinate plans with the juvenile's legal guardian as appropriate,
    b. arrange for a sufficient supply of current medications to last until the juvenile can be seen by a community health care professional, and
    c. for juveniles with critical medical, mental health, or dental needs, make arrangements or referrals for follow-up services with community clinicians.
2. All aspects of the standard are addressed by written policy and defined procedures.

Definition

Discharge planning refers to the process of providing sufficient medications and arranging for necessary follow-up health services before the juvenile's release to the community.

Discussion

The intent of this standard is that facility health care professionals ensure that patients' health needs are met during transition to a community health care professional.

Discharge planning includes the following: (1) formal linkages between the facility and community-based organizations, (2) lists of community health professionals, (3) discussions with the juvenile that emphasize the importance of appropriate follow-up and aftercare, and (4) specific appointments and medications that are arranged for the patient at the time of release.

Patients with a communicable disease or other serious medical or mental health conditions are given more than a list of community resources. Referrals are made to specialized clinics or community health professionals or, if appropriate, direct admission to a community hospital may be arranged.

Adequate discharge planning is contingent on timely notification by child care staff of the juvenile's scheduled release. However, if notification is not provided, health professionals still have a responsibility to ensure ongoing patient care with community health professionals. Follow-up care also may be required by public health laws (e.g., for active tuberculosis or sexually transmitted infections).

Optional Recommendations

The discharge process begins on admission and continues throughout the juvenile's incarceration. Close coordination is encouraged between designated health staff and any correctional, probation, or parole staff responsible for planning juvenile release. With the juvenile's permission, or that of the legal guardian where required, health staff may share necessary information and arrange for transfer of health summaries and relevant health records to community clinicians or others assisting in planning or providing for services on release.

Involving parents, if available, may help in the success of ongoing treatment. This is especially true for juveniles with chronic disease where education and counseling opportunities for the parents are included.

Programs where community health professionals contact juveniles in preparation for release are very effective, not only in providing the health services needed but also in fostering medication adherence. Some studies indicate that establishing therapeutic relationships with community health professionals before release and making formal preparations for return to the community that focus on transition issues also help reduce recidivism.

SECTION F – HEALTH PROMOTION

Y-F-01
important

HEALTHY LIFESTYLE PROMOTION

Standard

Health education is offered to all juveniles; individual health instruction is provided to all patients.

Compliance Indicators

1. The health record documents that patients receive individual health education and instruction in *self-care* for their health condition.
2. For general health education of juveniles, compliance requires, at a minimum, the availability of brochures and pamphlets on a variety of health topics in areas accessible to all juveniles (e.g., library, housing areas).
3. Educational programs are age specific.
4. All aspects of the standard are addressed by written policy and defined procedures.

Definitions

Health education is information on preventing illness and maintaining a healthy lifestyle.

Self-care is care for a condition that can be treated by the juvenile and may include over-the-counter medications.

Discussion

This standard intends to educate patients in self-care strategies and promote healthy lifestyle choices among all juveniles housed in the facility. The health education program may be provided by health staff, program staff, child care staff, or volunteers.

Patients can benefit from individual instruction in self-care and in ways to maintain their optimal health. In facilities with relatively short lengths of stay, this individual education may be the primary source of health education.

However, in addition to the one-to-one health teaching and counseling that may occur during health encounters, facilities are expected to provide opportunities for all juveniles to enhance their knowledge of health and healthy lifestyles. Facilities with specialized populations and those with relatively longer lengths of stay should provide a variety of resources and opportunities for learning about health-related topics. General health education methods may include classes, audio- and videotapes, and brochures and pamphlets. Brochures and pamphlets from various community-based organizations are readily available to facilities for distribution. Facilities with in-house video channels may use a video program on health matters to provide information.

Optional Recommendations

The following list contains some subjects for health education:
- alcohol and other drug problems;
- chronic diseases and disabilities;
- comprehensive family planning (including services and referrals);
- counseling in preparation for release;
- effects of smoking, use of tobacco products, and smoking cessation;
- hepatitis (A, B, and C);
- HIV infection and AIDS;
- immunizations;
- "keep-on-person" medications;
- nutrition;
- parenting skills;
- perinatal care;
- personal hygiene;
- physical fitness;
- prevention of sexual and other physical violence;
- preventive oral health care;
- self-examination for breast or testicular cancer;
- sexually transmitted infections;
- stress management; and
- tuberculosis.

Health staff can benefit from receiving training in the techniques and methods that are effective with juveniles. These may include motivational interactions, peer education initiatives, standard curriculum, and use of the creative arts.

Y-F-02
important

NUTRITION AND MEDICAL DIETS

Standard

Nutrition and medical diets are provided that enhance patients' health, and are modified when necessary to meet specific requirements related to clinical conditions.

Compliance Indicators

1. Regular and medical diets are nutritionally adequate and appropriate for age and gender groups.
2. Orders for medical diets include the type of diet, the duration for which it is to be provided, and special instructions, if any.
3. A registered or licensed dietitian reviews regular and medical diets for nutritional adequacy at least every 6 months and whenever a substantial change in the menus is made. Review may take place through a documented

on-site visit or by written consultation. Either way, written documentation of menu reviews includes the date, signature, and title of the consulting dietitian.

4. Workers who prepare regular and medical diets are trained in preparing the diets, including appropriate substitutions and portions.

5. When juveniles refuse prescribed diets, follow-up nutritional counseling is provided.

6. All aspects of the standard are addressed by written policy and defined procedures.

Definitions

Medical diets are special diets ordered for temporary or permanent health conditions that restrict the types, preparation, and/or amounts of food. Examples include restricted calorie, low sodium, low fat, pureed, soft, liquid, and nutritional supplementation diets. The medical diets addressed in this standard do not include special diets ordered for religious or security reasons.

A *heart-healthy diet* refers to foods that are low in saturated fat, cholesterol, and sodium and high in fiber as promoted by the American Heart Association.

Discussion

This standard intends that the food served will help juveniles be healthy, supplying adequate nutrition needed during different phases of growth and development, and meets the special dietary needs of those with health conditions.

The basic nutrition referred to in this standard is given to juveniles in segregation as well as to all others. Adequate nutrition, including medical diets, is provided during extended periods of lockdown.

Adolescents generally require more calories than adults and may require more frequent meals or snacks. Proper nutrition for adolescents has long-term positive effects on physical and emotional development. Dietitians should advise the responsible health authority on these issues on a regular basis, and be available for consultation to staff and juveniles alike.

Juveniles who fail to adhere to medical diets are not disciplined, but counseled. A decision to stop medical diets is a therapeutic decision.

Health staff should receive training in food–drug interactions, instruct patients accordingly, and prescribe diets as necessary. For example, caffeine makes a significant number of psychotropic medications less effective.

Optional Recommendations

Obesity is an increasing concern for juveniles and, until recently, not enough attention was given to the role the institutional food offerings may have in contributing to the problem. Facilities are encouraged to adopt a general *heart-healthy diet*. While this may substantially reduce the need for individual medical diets (e.g., diabetic, hypertensive), juveniles with certain health conditions (e.g., immunocompromised, organ failure) still require individual medical diets.

Y-F-03
important

EXERCISE

Standard

All juveniles are offered the health benefits of exercise.

Compliance Indicators

1. *Exercise* takes place outside the juvenile's room in an area large enough to accommodate the activity.
2. Exercise is offered to all custody classes of juveniles except those in transient status or lockdown for a week or less.
3. The frequency of exercise is at least 1hour daily, 7 days a week.
4. All aspects of the standard are addressed by written policy and defined procedures.

Definition

Exercise is increased aerobic activity that stimulates and improves physical and mental health through the use of large-muscle activities such as walking, jogging in place, basketball, and isometrics.

Discussion

An intent of this standard is to improve juveniles' overall health through exercise. For adolescents, recreation is necessary for the proper development of the body. High-energy activities also help alleviate stress that may build up among adolescents. Recreational exercise can improve cardiovascular performance and enhance overall physical and mental health. Exercise can be helpful in controlling anxiety, nervousness, manic episodes, and depression.

Regarding the use of outside yards, gymnasia, and multipurpose rooms, providing opportunities for exercise (e.g., basketball, handball, running, calisthenics) satisfies the standard even if juveniles do not take advantage of them. Although such activities may be more productive under the supervision of a recreational staff person, this is not required.

Permitting in-room exercises does not constitute compliance with standard.

Optional Recommendations

Health staff, including mental health staff, should encourage patients under their care to take advantage of exercise opportunities.

There should be a designated room or area (inside or outside) for exercise. Daily outdoor exercise, whenever possible, is recommended. It is also recommended that health staff advise facility staff about health risks of strenuous exercise during inclement environmental conditions (e.g., extreme heat or cold). Likewise, health staff should alert facility staff when there are safety problems with recreational equipment or the environment used for recreation.

Y-F-04
important

PERSONAL HYGIENE

Standard

The facility provides sufficient services and supplies so that juveniles' personal hygiene needs are met.

Compliance Indicators

1. In every area where juveniles are detained for at least 48 hours, there is a tub or a shower with hot and cold running water.
2. All custody classes of juveniles have the opportunity to shower daily.
3. Personal hygiene items include minimally:
   a. soap,
   b. comb,
   c. soft round-bristle toothbrush,
   d. toothpaste,
   e. deodorant,
   f. toilet paper, and
   g. in facilities housing females, sanitary napkins and tampons.
4. Haircuts and individual shaving instruments are available.
5. Juveniles receive a change of outer clothing three times a week, a daily change of underwear, and a weekly bed linen and towel change.
6. Shower, bath, and laundry facilities are in good working order.
7. All aspects of the standard are addressed by written policy and defined procedures.

Discussion

An intent of this standard is that all juveniles have the opportunity to maintain their personal hygiene.

All juveniles, including those in any type of segregation or special housing, are able to care for their personal hygiene. Daily schedules should include sufficient time for showering without excessive haste. Those on suicide watch, in the infirmary, or in special medical or mental health housing are provided with the same opportunities for personal care unless there is a specific medical order to the contrary.

Personal hygiene practices can be particularly beneficial for those experiencing mental health difficulties or substance abuse problems. For many patients, self-esteem is enhanced as hygiene improves. On the other hand, lack of attention to personal hygiene may be an important predictor of impending mental illness. Patients with severe psychiatric disturbances, active depression, or significant intellectual deficits may not pay attention to their personal hygiene.

Optional Recommendations

Health staff should offer classes in personal hygiene as part of the health promotion initiative (see Y-F-01 Healthy Lifestyle Promotion). Juveniles with chronic medical problems (e.g., diabetes, ostomies or shunts, chronic skin disease) that present challenges to maintaining good hygiene should be given assistance in learning how to cope with their specific needs. Mental health and child care staff should assist juveniles in maintaining appropriate personal hygiene that improves mental well-being.

It is recommended that facilities consider the use of nonslip materials in shower areas.

Y-F-05
important

USE OF TOBACCO

Standard

The facility is smoke-free for juveniles and staff, and juveniles may not use tobacco in any form. There are prevention and abatement activities regarding the use of all tobacco products.

Compliance Indicators

1. For juveniles, smoking is prohibited and tobacco may not be used in any form.
2. For staff, smoking is prohibited inside the building; smoking outside occurs only in designated areas.
3. At a minimum, the prevention and abatement program includes appropriate pharmaceutical support for withdrawal when medically indicated, and written materials on prevention and abatement of tobacco use. The written materials are available in areas accessible to all juveniles (e.g., clinic, library, housing).

4.   All aspects of the standard are addressed by written policy and defined procedures.

Discussion

This standard intends that juveniles, staff, and visitors are not exposed to the detrimental effects of tobacco products.

Recognizing the evidence that the use of all tobacco products and exposure to second-hand smoke are dangerous to health, prevention and abatement efforts are undertaken. These efforts include health education classes, video- and audiotapes, and self-help and other smoking cessation aids such as the availability of nicotine replacement products. Organizations such as the American Cancer Society, the American Lung Association, and the American Heart Association have resources to help facilities develop prevention and education programs.

Given the long-term negative effects of smoking on health, special efforts are taken to help adolescents who smoke.

Optional Recommendations

No facility should be involved in the manufacture of cigarettes or other tobacco products.

Some chronically mentally ill patients use smoking to control anxiety and other symptoms. These individuals should receive special management in a nonsmoking environment.

SECTION G – SPECIAL NEEDS AND SERVICES

Y-G-01
essential

CHRONIC DISEASE SERVICES

Standard

Patients with *chronic diseases* are identified and enrolled in a *chronic disease program* to decrease the frequency and severity of the symptoms, prevent disease progression and complication, and improve function.

Compliance Indicators

1. The responsible physician establishes and annually approves clinical protocols consistent with *national clinical practice guidelines*. These clinical protocols for the management of chronic diseases include, but are not limited to, the following:
    a. asthma,
    b. attention deficit hyperactivity disorder (ADHD),
    c. diabetes,
    d. HIV,
    e. seizure disorder,
    f. major mental illness, and
    g. tuberculosis disease or infection.
2. Documentation in the health record confirms that clinicians are following chronic disease protocols by:
    a. determining the frequency of follow-up for medical evaluation;
    b. adjusting treatment modality as clinically indicated;
    c. indicating the type and frequency of diagnostic testing and therapeutic regimens;
    d. writing appropriate instructions for diet, exercise, adaptation to the correctional environment, and medication; and
    e. clinically justifying any deviation from the protocol.
3. The responsible physician annually approves the chronic disease protocols.
4. The responsible physician implements a system to ensure continuity of medications for chronic diseases.
5. Chronic illnesses are listed on the master problem list.
6. The facility maintains a list of chronic care patients.
7. All aspects of the standard are addressed by written policy and defined procedures.

Definitions

The National Academy of Sciences' Institute of Medicine defines *clinical practice guidelines* as systematically developed, science-based statements designed to assist clinician and patient with decisions about appropriate health care for specific clinical circumstances. Clinical practice guidelines are used to assist clinical decision making, assess and ensure the quality of care, provide education about clinical disease, guide the allocation of health care resources, and reduce the risk of legal liability for negligent care.

National clinical practice guidelines are those presented by national professional organizations and accepted by experts in the respective medical field. (NCCHC's clinical guidelines are available at www.ncchc.org.)

Chronic disease is an illness or condition that affects an individual's well-being for an extended interval, usually at least 6 months, and generally is not curable but can be managed to provide optimum functioning within any limitations the condition imposes on the individual.

The *chronic disease program* incorporates a treatment plan and regular clinic visits. The clinician monitors the patient's progress during clinic visits and, when necessary, changes the treatment. The program also includes patient education for symptom management.

Discussion

This standard intends that patients with chronic diseases are properly managed.

Studies have found that correctional facilities house a significant number of juveniles with chronic disease. Nationally recognized, generally accepted clinical guidelines exist for many diseases common in correctional populations. These guidelines help clinicians to practice the best medicine aimed at improving patient outcomes. For patients whose disease is well controlled, the guidelines help to maintain good health and avoid unnecessary treatment.

Success in minimizing symptoms is best achieved through health professional–patient teamwork in understanding what is needed regarding medications, patient education, monitoring, and environmental controls.

Patients with chronic diseases benefit from regular clinic visits for evaluation and management by health care clinicians. By reviewing the patient's history and progress over time, the clinician can optimize the treatment plan. In contrast, an episodic approach (which is not recommended) can lead to increased morbidity, mortality, and cost. Without tracking patients' progress (or lack thereof), the patient's health can deteriorate rapidly.

The use of flow sheets facilitates tracking these patients.

Optional Recommendations

In the treatment of chronic diseases, the best system would be one in which patients are seen based on chronic care protocols addressing total disease management. This requires clear indicators of the severity of the patient's condition and whether the condition is stable, improving, or deteriorating. Relevant baseline laboratory and other testing data should be obtained and recorded in the patient's health record. Patients with chronic disease should be enrolled in an appropriate program for the management of their disease.

For juveniles enrolled in an HIV program, care should be supervised by an HIV specialist who will initiate and change therapeutic regimens as medically indicated. Teaching juveniles how to cope with the disease and help prevent complications is valuable for successful transition to community care. The parent or guardian of the juvenile will also benefit from education about the disease. Confidentiality issues and the patient's wishes should be considered along with the legal requirements of the jurisdiction.

The management of chronic care patients should be monitored through the facility's continuous quality improvement (CQI) process. (See Appendix C – Continuous Quality Improvement.)

Y-G-02
essential

PATIENTS WITH SPECIAL HEALTH NEEDS

Standard

A proactive program exists that provides care for *special needs patients* who require close medical supervision or multidisciplinary care.

Compliance Indicators

1. Individual *treatment plans* are developed by a physician or other qualified clinician at the time the condition is identified and updated when warranted.
2. The treatment plan includes, at a minimum:
   a. the frequency of follow-up for medical and mental health evaluation and adjustment of treatment modality,
   b. the type and frequency of diagnostic testing and therapeutic regimens, and
   c. when appropriate, instructions about diet, exercise, adaptation to the correctional environment, and medication.
3. Special needs are listed on the master problem list.
4. The facility maintains a list of special needs patients.
5. All aspects of the standard are addressed by written policy and defined procedures.

Definitions

Special needs patients include those with chronic diseases or conditions that require regular care. Examples of special needs patients and their conditions are provided below.

Developmentally disabled individuals include those with limited intellectual ability who may need habilitation planning, assistance in accepting the limitations of their conditions, and special attention to their physical safety in the corrections environment.

Dialysis patients are those with end-stage renal disease requiring hemodialysis or peritoneal dialysis on a recurrent basis.

Fragile juveniles include those who suffer from conditions that impair their ability to function to the extent that they require assistance in activities of daily living (e.g., dressing, feeding, transferring, toileting).

Physical disabilities can refer to mobility impairments (e.g., amputations, paraplegia) or to other disabilities that limit daily functioning (e.g., visual, hearing, or speech impairments).

For *pregnant juveniles,* refer to standards Y-G-07 Care of the Pregnant Juvenile and Y-G-09 Family Planning Services.

Serious communicable diseases include those transmitted sexually, through the respiratory system, or by infected blood (e.g., syphilis, gonorrhea, chlamydia, HIV, tuberculosis, hepatitis).

Patients with *serious mental health* needs include those with basic psychotic disorders or mood disorders (e.g., manic-depressives), self-mutilators, the aggressive mentally ill, those with posttraumatic stress disorders, and suicidal juveniles.

For *terminally ill* juveniles, refer to standard Y-G-11 Care for the Terminally Ill.

A *treatment plan* is a series of written statements specifying a patient's particular course of therapy and the roles of qualified health care professionals in carrying it out.

Discussion

This standard intends to ensure that juveniles with significant health conditions receive ongoing multidisciplinary care.

The special needs program serves a broad range of health conditions and problems that require the physician or other designated qualified health care professionals to design a treatment plan tailored to the patient's needs. The treatment plan is individualized, typically multidisciplinary, and based on an assessment of the patient's needs, and includes a statement of short- and long-term goals as well as the methods by which these goals will be pursued. When clinically indicated, the treatment plan gives patients access to the range of supportive and rehabilitative services (e.g., physical therapy, individual or group counseling, self-help groups) that the treating clinician deems appropriate.

Patients with special needs are followed closely. Regularly scheduled chronic clinics are a good way to ensure continuity of care. The master problem list includes known drug allergies and any special needs. The use of flow sheets facilitates tracking these patients, particularly those with chronic illnesses. The parameters to be followed on the flow sheets coincide with criteria established for each of the common chronic illnesses, thereby facilitating review for compliance with the criteria in standard Y-A-06 Continuous Quality Improvement Program. (See also Y-G-01 Chronic Disease Services.)

Health professionals should be aware that many patients with mental illness also have co-occurring substance abuse disorders. In addition, posttraumatic stress disorders also are common problems among juveniles due to past sexual, physical, or emotional abuse. Alcohol and other substance abuse also can be significant problems requiring individual treatment planning.

The treatment plan may use any format that contains all of the required elements. Specific individual treatment forms are preferable since they facilitate developing a comprehensive plan that is easily identifiable. SOAP (subjective, objective, assessment, plan) notation in the progress notes is another way to document a treatment plan.

Optional Recommendations

Treatment plans for patients with mental health conditions should incorporate ways to address the patients' problems and enhance patients' strengths, involve patients in their development, and include relapse prevention risk management strategies. The strategies should describe signs and symptoms associated with relapse or recurring difficulties (e.g., auditory hallucinations), how the patient thinks a relapse can be averted, and how best to help the patient manage crises.

Treatment plans for the developmentally disabled may focus on helping the juvenile to cope with the correctional environment and alerting child care staff to the special needs of the juvenile. Developmental disabilities have implications for health education, informed consent issues, and the manner in which the juvenile may perceive and respond to verbal communication from child care staff. Juveniles with intellectual limitations are prone to become victims in the correctional environment and may need special housing arrangements.

A treatment plan should be developed or revised for any juvenile expressing suicidal ideation. This treatment plan should be developed by the mental health staff in conjunction with the patient to address relapse prevention and initiate a risk management plan. The risk management plan should describe signs, symptoms, and the circumstances in which the risk for suicide is likely to recur; how recurrence of suicidal thoughts can be avoided; and actions the patient or staff can take if suicidal thoughts do occur.

Performance Measures

1. In 100% of the cases where a juvenile requires a special needs treatment plan and good clinical practice would ordinarily result in a decrease of symptom severity or frequency, quarterly reviews of the juvenile's progress shows deceasing severity or frequency of related symptoms.
2. Quarterly review of clinical progress of juveniles who require a special needs treatment plan confirms decreasing numbers of events requiring emergency intervention.

Performance Measure Expectations

The expectation is that the performance measures are met 100% of the time.

The responsible health authority decides what methods of study and documentation are to be used in internal reviews to assess compliance with these measures. All such studies and tracking methods are incorporated into the facility's CQI program.

Measures #1 and #2 both require a specific periodic record review process to track the issues, first on an individual level and then on aggregate data to reflect trends of treatment outcome.

Y-G-03
essential

INFIRMARY CARE

Standard

Infirmary care, when provided, is appropriate to meet the serious needs of patients.

Compliance Indicators

1. Policy defines the scope of medical, psychiatric, and nursing care provided in the *infirmary* setting.
2. Patients are always *within sight or hearing* of a qualified health care professional.
3. The number of sufficient and appropriate qualified health care professionals in the infirmary is determined based on the number of patients, the severity of their illnesses, and the level of care required for each.
4. A supervising registered nurse is on site at least once every 24 hours.
5. A manual of nursing care procedures is consistent with the state's nurse practice act and licensing requirements.
6. Admission to and discharge from infirmary care occur only on the order of a physician (or other clinician where permitted by virtue of his or her credentials and scope of practice).

7. The frequency of physician and nursing rounds in the infirmary is specified based on the categories of care provided.
8. A complete inpatient health record is kept for each patient and includes:
    a. admitting order that includes the admitting diagnosis, medication, diet, activity restrictions, diagnostic tests required, and frequency of vital sign monitoring and other follow-up;
    b. complete documentation of the care and treatment given;
    c. the medication administration record; and
    d. a discharge plan and discharge notes.
9. If the inpatient record is retained separately from the outpatient record, a copy of the discharge summary from infirmary care is placed in the patient's outpatient chart.
10. All aspects of the standard are addressed by written policy and defined procedures.

Definitions

Infirmary care is care provided to patients with an illness or diagnosis that requires daily monitoring, medication and/or therapy, or assistance with activities of daily living at a level needing skilled nursing intervention.

An *infirmary* is an area in the facility accommodating patients for a period of 24 hours or more, expressly set up and operated for the purpose of caring for patients who need skilled nursing care but do not need hospitalization or placement in a licensed nursing facility, and whose care cannot be managed safely in an outpatient setting. It is not the area itself but the scope of care provided that makes the bed an infirmary bed.

Within sight or hearing of a qualified health care professional means that the patient can gain the professional's attention through visual or auditory signals. Call lights and buzzer systems can be useful ways to ensure this. The use of nonmedical staff to alert health staff in the event of need does not constitute compliance.

Observation beds are beds designated for medical or mental observation for specific purposes, such as watching the patient's response to a change in medication regimen. Patients also can be placed in observation beds to prevent them from eating or drinking before a medical test that requires such restriction, to allow patients to recover from day surgeries or medical procedures, or to watch the general behavior of juveniles whose mental stability appears questionable.

Sheltered housing, as opposed to infirmary or observation beds, provides a protective environment that does not require 24-hour nursing care. The beds can be in the infirmary itself or in other designated areas (e.g., where hospice-level care or "step-down" or transitional mental health care is provided). Sheltered housing is equivalent to home care for those not confined to an institutional setting.

Discussion

This standard intends to establish the principles and practices for infirmary care in the facility.

Patients admitted to the infirmary can be classified into two bed categories: infirmary care and *observation*. Procedures or individual treatment plans must specify the frequency of nursing and physician rounds for each category of individuals housed in the infirmary.

1. Infirmary care patients are admitted and discharged only on a physician's order (or by another clinician where permitted by virtue of his or her credentials and scope of practice).
2. Observation patients may be placed by a qualified health care professional other than a physician; however, a physician's order is needed to keep them longer than 24 hours.

The inpatient record includes the admitting notes, a discharge plan (see Y-E-12 Continuity of Care During Incarceration) including a summary when the patient is discharged, and complete documentation of the care and treatment given.

Patients may be admitted to infirmaries for psychiatric care. When admitted for mental health reasons, the patient's mental health care is supervised by mental health clinicians. Facilities may offer medical and psychiatric infirmary care in one infirmary or have two separate, dedicated areas. In either situation, the psychiatric infirmary care is subject to the requirements of this standard.

Some facilities provide *sheltered housing* for juveniles whose health needs require a more protective environment than that in the general housing areas. Sheltered housing beds may or may not be in the infirmary area. The requirements of this standard do not apply to sheltered housing beds since these individuals are not inpatients.

Optional Recommendation

Enhancement of quality care in the infirmary begins with assigning program responsibility to one physician and a registered nurse manager. Depending on the size of the infirmary, this physician may be employed full or part time.

Y-G-04
essential

BASIC MENTAL HEALTH SERVICES

Standard

Mental health services are available for all juveniles who require them.

Compliance Indicators

1. Treatment services minimally include on- or off-site crisis intervention including short-term individual and group therapy follow-up, as needed, and psychotropic medication management.
2. Mental health, medical, and substance abuse services are sufficiently coordinated such that patient management is appropriately integrated, health needs are met, and the impact of any of these conditions on each other is adequately addressed.
3. All aspects of the standard are addressed by written policy and defined procedures.

Definition

Mental health services include the use of a variety of psychosocial and pharmacological therapies, either individual or group, including biological, psychological, and social, to alleviate symptoms, attain appropriate functioning, and prevent relapse.

Discussion

This standard intends that juveniles with mental health problems are able to maintain their best level of functioning.

In the correctional setting, as in most other environments, the immediate objective of mental health treatment is to alleviate symptoms of serious mental disorders and prevent relapses to sustain patients' ability to function safely in their environment. Mental health treatment is more than prescribing psychotropic medications. Treatment goals include the development of self-understanding, self-improvement, and skills to cope with and overcome disabilities associated with various mental disorders.

Crisis intervention and provision of appropriate psychotropic medications are also expected for juveniles with short lengths of stay and in facilities that transfer juveniles with serious mental health problems to other facilities. Facilities housing significant numbers of mental health patients with longer lengths of stay are expected to offer more extensive mental health programming. Correctional facilities that provide for the needs of patients requiring psychiatric hospitalization levels of care are expected to mirror treatment provided in inpatient settings in the community.

For further guidance in providing services, see *Psychiatric Services in Jails and Prisons*, Second Edition (American Psychiatric Association) and *Standards for Psychology Services in Jails, Prisons, Correctional Facilities, and Agencies*, Third Edition (International Association for Correctional and Forensic Psychology). NCCHC's *Standards for Mental Health Services in Correctional Facilities* may be especially helpful.

See also Y-G-02 Patients With Special Health Needs, Y-G-05 Suicide Prevention Program, and Y-G-08 Juveniles With Alcohol and Other Drug Problems.

Optional Recommendations

The use of an integrated and multidisciplinary team (including child care staff) to develop treatment plans for juveniles displaying manipulative behavior can be effective. These treatment plans should include behavioral contracts with the patient to reinforce positive behavior.

For patients treated previously in the community, the responsible health authority should obtain necessary records from community mental health clinicians.

Y-G-05
essential

SUICIDE PREVENTION PROGRAM

Standard

The facility staff identifies suicidal juveniles and intervenes appropriately.

Compliance Indicators

1. A suicide prevention program includes the following outcomes:
    a. facility staff identify suicidal juveniles and immediately initiate precautions,
    b. suicidal juveniles are evaluated promptly by the designated health professional who directs the intervention and ensures follow-up as needed,
    c. *actively suicidal* juveniles are placed on constant observation, and
    d. *potentially suicidal* juveniles are monitored on an irregular schedule with no more than 15 minutes between two checks. If, however, the potentially suicidal juvenile is placed in isolation, constant observation is required.
2. Key components of a suicide prevention program include the following:
    a. training,
    b. identification,
    c. referral,
    d. evaluation,
    e. treatment,
    f. housing and monitoring,

  g. communication,

  h. intervention,

  i. notification,

  j. review, and

  k. debriefing.

3. The use of other juveniles in any way (e.g., companions, suicide-prevention aides) is not a substitute for staff supervision.

4. Treatment plans addressing suicidal ideation and its reoccurrence are developed, and patient follow-up occurs as clinically indicated.

5. The responsible health authority approves the suicide prevention plan; training curriculum for staff, intake screening for suicide potential and referral protocols; and training for staff conducting the suicide screening at intake.

6. All aspects of the standard are addressed by written policy and defined procedures.

Definitions

Actively suicidal juveniles express a state of acute thought of completing suicide associated with imminent risk. They should be placed on constant observation.

Potentially suicidal juveniles are not actively suicidal but express suicidal ideation and/or have a recent history of self-destructive behavior. They should be observed at staggered intervals not to exceed every 15 minutes (e.g., 5, 10, 7 minutes).

Discussion

This standard is intended to ensure that suicides are prevented if at all possible. When suicides do occur, appropriate corrective action is identified and implemented to prevent future suicides. While juveniles may become suicidal at any point during their stay, high-risk periods include immediately upon admission; after adjudication, after return to a facility from court; after the receipt of bad news regarding self or family (e.g., serious illness, the loss of a loved one); prolonged stays in juvenile detention facilities; or after suffering humiliation (e.g., sexual assault) or rejection. Juveniles entering or unable to cope with segregation, other specialized single-room housing assignments, or room confinements (e.g., time-out, quiet time, separation, etc.) are at high risk for suicide. In addition, juveniles who are in the early stages of recovery from severe depression may be at risk. Recent research points out that adolescent suicides in correctional settings have different high-risk periods compared to adults.

Key components of a suicide prevention program include the following:

1. Training. All staff members who work with juveniles are trained to recognize verbal and behavioral cues that indicate potential suicide and how to

respond appropriately. Initial and at least biennial training are provided, although annual training is highly recommended.

2. Identification. The receiving screening form contains observation and interview items related to potential suicide risk. If a staff member identifies someone who is potentially suicidal, the juvenile is placed on suicide precautions and is referred immediately to mental health staff.

3. Referral. There are procedures for referring potentially suicidal juveniles and those who have attempted suicide to mental health care clinicians or facilities. The procedures specify a time frame for response to the referral.

4. Evaluation. An evaluation, conducted by a qualified mental health professional, determines the level of suicide risk, level of supervision needed, and need for transfer to an inpatient mental health facility or program. Patients are reassessed regularly to identify any change in condition indicating a need for a change in supervision level or required transfer or commitment. The evaluation includes procedures for periodic follow-up assessment after the individual's discharge from suicide precautions.

5. Treatment. Strategies and services to address the underlying reasons (e.g., depression, auditory commands) for the juvenile's suicide ideation are to be considered. The strategies include treatment needs when the patient is at heightened risk to suicide as well as follow-up treatment interventions and monitoring strategies to reduce the likelihood of relapse.

6. Housing and Monitoring. Unless constant supervision is maintained, a suicidal juvenile is not isolated but is housed in the general population, mental health unit, or medical infirmary, and located in close proximity to staff. All cells or rooms housing suicidal juveniles are as suicide-resistant as possible (e.g., without protrusions that would enable hanging). There are procedures for monitoring a juvenile identified as potentially suicidal and juveniles are monitored on an irregular schedule with no more than 15 minutes between two checks. Although several protocols exist for monitoring suicidal juveniles, any actively suicidal juvenile (either threatening or engaging in self-injurious behavior) should be observed by a staff member on a continuous, uninterrupted basis. Other supervision aids (e.g., closed circuit television) can be used as a supplement to, but never as a substitute for, staff monitoring.

7. Communication. Procedures for communication between mental health care, health care, and child care staff regarding juvenile status are in place to provide clear and current information. These procedures include communication between transferring authorities (e.g., local court system, county facility, medical/psychiatric facility) and facility child care staff.

8. Intervention. There are procedures addressing how to handle a suicide attempt in progress, including appropriate first-aid measures.

9. Notification. Procedures state when correctional administrators, outside authorities, and family members are notified of potential, attempted, or completed suicides.

10. Reporting. Procedures for documenting the identification and monitoring of potential or attempted suicides are detailed, as are procedures for reporting a completed suicide.

11. Review. There are procedures for mental health, medical, and administrative review if a suicide or a serious suicide attempt (as defined by the suicide plan) occurs. See Y-A-10 Procedure in the Event of a Juvenile Death for details.

12. Debriefing. There are procedures for offering timely debriefing to all affected personnel and juveniles. Debriefing is a process whereby individuals are given an opportunity to express their thoughts and feelings about an incident (e.g., suicide or attempt), develop an understanding of stress symptoms resulting from the incident, and develop ways to deal with those symptoms. Debriefing can be done by an in-house response team or outside consultants prepared to handle these highly stressful situations. There are different approaches to the debriefing process, including some highly confrontational or "forced interventions" methods. Such methods are not intended under this standard.

A psychological autopsy for each suicide should be completed within 30 days. The typical psychological autopsy is based on a detailed review of all file information on the juvenile, a careful examination of the suicide site, and interviews with staff, juveniles, and family members familiar with the deceased. (See Y-A-10 Procedure in the Event of a Juvenile Death).

Optional Recommendations

Because suicide is a leading cause of death in juvenile facilities nationwide, an active approach to the management of suicidal juveniles is recommended. In facilities where 24-hour mental health staff coverage is not present, designated health and/or child care staff should be able to initiate suicide precautions until the mental health clinician on call can be contacted for further orders. On the other hand, only designated qualified mental health care professionals should be authorized to remove a juvenile from suicide precautionary measures.

Where feasible, persons trained in debriefing procedures should be used. Practical guidelines on the debriefing process are available from organizations such as the International Critical Incident Stress Foundation.

It is recommended that "cutting tools" be routinely issued to all staff or at least be readily available in all areas of the facility. These devices have been designed to be safe but effective instruments for interrupting a suicide by hanging.

Performance Measure

1. A continuous quality improvement (CQI) root cause analysis is conducted for all suicides and suicide attempts.

2. Remedial action is taken on identified policy, staff performance, environment, or other system failures that allowed the event to occur. The remedial change(s) are successful in preventing opportunities for future suicide attempts.

Performance Measure Expectations

The expectation is that the performance measures are met 100% of the time.

The responsible health authority decides what methods of study and documentation are to be used in internal reviews to assess compliance with these measures. All such studies and tracking methods are incorporated into the facility's CQI program.

Each serious suicide attempt or success, by required policy and procedures, is studied and reviewed on several levels already. This measure, which summarizes established procedures, requires that aggregate data be gathered and reviewed so that the success of identifying potentially suicidal juveniles and preventing their acting on suicidal impulses and thoughts can be confirmed or enhanced.

Y-G-06
essential

INTOXICATION AND WITHDRAWAL

Standard

Protocols exist for juveniles under the influence of alcohol or other drugs and those undergoing withdrawal.

Compliance Indicators

1. Established protocols are followed for the treatment and observation of individuals manifesting symptoms of intoxication or withdrawal.
2. The protocols are approved by the responsible physician, are current, and are consistent with nationally accepted guidelines.
3. *Detoxification* is done only under physician supervision in accordance with local, state, and federal laws.
4. Juveniles experiencing severe, life-threatening intoxication (overdose) or withdrawal are transferred immediately to a licensed acute care facility.
5. Individuals at risk for progression to more severe levels of intoxication or withdrawal are kept under constant observation by qualified health care professionals or health-trained child care staff, and when severe withdrawal symptoms are observed, a physician is consulted promptly.
6. If a pregnant juvenile is admitted with a history of *opiate* use (including the partial agonist buprenorphine), consultation occurs among the facility physician, the OB/GYN specialist treating the patient, and an opioid dependence treatment specialist so that the opiate dependence can be assessed and treated appropriately.

7. A policy addresses the management of juveniles, including pregnant juveniles, on methadone or similar substances. Juveniles entering the facility on such substances have their therapy continued, or a plan for appropriate treatment of the methadone withdrawal syndrome is initiated.
8. All aspects of the standard are addressed by written policy and defined procedures.

Definitions

Detoxification is the process by which an individual is gradually withdrawn from a drug by the administration of decreasing doses of the drug on which the person is physiologically dependent, of one that is cross-tolerant to it, or of one that medical research has demonstrated to be effective.

Opiates are any preparation or derivative of opium, as well as opioid, a synthetic narcotic that resembles an opiate in action but is not derived from opium.

Discussion

An intent of this standard is that juveniles who are intoxicated or undergoing withdrawal are properly managed.

Significant percentages of juveniles admitted to correctional facilities have a history of alcohol and/or other drug abuse. Newly incarcerated individuals may enter intoxicated or develop symptoms of drug withdrawal. Juveniles are at highest risk from PCP and crack cocaine intoxication. Barbiturate withdrawal, while less commonly seen in correctional settings, also may be life-threatening. Mild to moderate forms of withdrawal can worsen without appropriate treatment, and continued assessment is required.

The treatment for most non-life-threatening withdrawal is amelioration of symptoms, which can be managed in the convalescent or outpatient setting. Abstinence syndromes in certain groups (including those who are psychotic, epileptic, pregnant, or otherwise medically ill) may require different protocols. For example, current medical thinking is that pregnant patients should not be withdrawn from a methadone maintenance program.

History alone is not sufficient to determine the level of risk; vital signs and clinical status must be evaluated. Severe withdrawal syndromes should never be managed outside of a hospital. Deaths from acute intoxication or severe withdrawal have occurred in correctional facilities. In determining the level of symptoms that can be managed safely at the facility, the responsible physician must take into account the level of medical supervision that is available at all times.

Training for child care workers includes recognizing the signs and symptoms of intoxication and withdrawal (see Y-C-04 Health Training for Child Care Staff). Intoxication and withdrawal also present an increased potential for suicide, a factor that is to be incorporated into the training for staff as part of the suicide prevention program. When alcohol or other drug withdrawal occurs, a juvenile will be agitated and at higher risk for self-destructive behaviors.

Optional Recommendation

Resources that the responsible health authority can use to develop policies, train staff, and obtain further information include the American Society of Addiction Medicine and the American Academy of Addiction Psychiatry.

Y-G-07
essential

CARE OF THE PREGNANT JUVENILE

Standard

Pregnant juveniles receive timely and appropriate prenatal care, specialized obstetrical services when indicated, and postpartum care.

Compliance Indicators

1. Prenatal care includes:
   a. medical examinations,
   b. laboratory and diagnostic tests (including offering HIV testing and prophylaxis for the infant of the infected juvenile when indicated), and
   c. advice on appropriate levels of activity, safety precautions, and nutritional guidance and counseling.
2. A list of specialized obstetrical services is maintained.
3. There is a written agreement with a community facility for delivery.
4. There is documentation of appropriate postpartum care.
5. A list is kept of all pregnancies and their outcomes.
6. All aspects of the standard are addressed by written policy and defined procedures.

Discussion

This standard intends that the health of the pregnant juvenile and fetus are protected.

Before incarceration, many female juveniles have unhealthy lifestyles, including a history of using tobacco, alcohol, and other drugs extensively, and lack prenatal care. Therefore, many pregnancies can be classified as high risk. Other factors also complicate high-risk pregnancies, such as a positive HIV status, other sexually transmitted infections, malnutrition, obesity, adolescence, and increased anxiety, stress, and depression. As a result, specialized obstetrical staff, equipment, and other resources are often needed.

See also Y-A-08 Communication on Patients With Special Needs, Y-G-02 Patients With Special Health Needs, and Y-G-06 Intoxication and Withdrawal.

Optional Recommendations

Pregnant juveniles can benefit from educational programs focusing on self-care and parenting skills. Many communities have agencies that can assist with health education programs (e.g., county health departments, specialty clinics, local hospitals). Such resources should be used.

Documentation of the patient's prenatal history should accompany her to the hospital.

Generally, psychotropic medications have deleterious effects on the developing fetus. Therefore, mental health staff should consult with medical staff regarding the potential effects of any prescribed psychotropics on the fetus, as well as the mother's need for continuing medication.

Postpartum depression may manifest itself in different ways, particularly when the adolescent mother is incarcerated and separated from her newborn immediately after birth. Medical staff, therefore, work with the mental health staff to address the issue and provide appropriate treatment.

Pregnancy care and outcomes should be monitored through the continuous quality improvement process at least annually.

Y-G-08
important

JUVENILES WITH ALCOHOL AND OTHER DRUG PROBLEMS

Standard

Juveniles with alcohol or other drug (AOD) problems are assessed and properly managed by a physician or, where permitted by law, other qualified health care professionals.

Compliance Indicators

1. There are written clinical guidelines for the management of AOD patients.
2. Disorders associated with AOD (e.g., HIV, liver disease) are recognized and treated.
3. The child care staff are trained in recognizing intoxication problems in juveniles and discussing AOD problems with them.
4. There is evidence of communication and coordination between medical, mental health, and substance abuse staff regarding AOD care.

5. There is on-site individual counseling, group therapy, or self-help groups.
6. Didactic approaches to drug education are available.
7. All aspects of the standard are addressed by written policy and defined procedures.

Discussion

The standard intends that juveniles are provided with the opportunity to address their addictions. Effective intervention in adolescence may result in drug-free adulthood and lifelong abstinence.

All health care professionals can have a part in treating the diseases of alcohol and other drug abuse. Health staff have several roles in this regard: (1) appropriate assessment of intoxication and withdrawal (see Y-G-06 Intoxication and Withdrawal), (2) treatment of disorders associated with AOD (e.g., HIV, liver disease), (3) appropriate prescription of psychoactive drugs as required (see Y-G-04 Basic Mental Health Services), and (4) supportive and appropriate motivational counseling during clinical encounters. Inquiry about and support of the patient's efforts to deal with AOD problems by the clinician is often a strong motivator.

Ideally, individual counseling, group counseling, self-help groups, residential programs, and clinical management are coordinated. In any event, policy and procedures define the roles of the AOD treatment team and the health care team, as well as the areas of mutual interest and collaboration. Clinical management of the patient is supervised by a physician. Community self-help initiatives such as Alcoholics Anonymous, Alateen, and Narcotics Anonymous may be appropriate supplements or alternatives to counseling provided by in-house staff.

Optional Recommendations

Patients with AOD disorders present special challenges in diagnosis and treatment, and their physicians should have relevant special training.

Counselors who treat AOD problems should be properly qualified to do so by a recognized accrediting body. Medical and mental health clinicians can facilitate treatment by referring juveniles for treatment, providing counseling to motivate juveniles to receive treatment, legitimizing self-help groups, tailoring controlled substances prescribing practices, and otherwise being a partner in the process of treatment.

Juveniles commonly have the co-occurring disorders of mental illness and substance abuse. Ideally, they will be treated by clinicians who are trained in both disciplines. Mental health subspecialties often have differing therapeutic approaches that need to be modified when treating patients with co-occurring disorders. Additionally, a patient's functional and organic needs often require a holistic approach by medical and mental health professionals. A team approach also facilitates communication among professionals.

Y-G-09
important

FAMILY PLANNING SERVICES

Standard

The facility provides comprehensive family planning services, in accordance with state statutes, on the premises or by referral; pregnant juveniles have access to services as they would in the community.

Compliance Indicator

1. Pregnant juveniles are given comprehensive counseling and assistance, consistent with local laws, in accordance with their expressed desires regarding their pregnancy, whether they elect to keep the child, use adoption services, or have an abortion.
2. Counseling and social services regarding all aspects of sexuality should be available in the facility or by referral to appropriate community agencies for both males and females.
3. All aspects of the standard are addressed by written policy and defined procedures.

Discussion

This standard intends that all juveniles are educated and prepared for responsible sexual behavior, including preparation for parenthood and parenting skills; pregnant juveniles receive services as they would in the community.

Incarceration of sexually active juveniles often prevents access to appropriate family planning services. Educational printed materials should be age appropriate and in the primary languages spoken in the community. Contraceptive publications should be available for both males and females; contraceptive materials should be available upon discharge from the facility.

Pregnancy detection and counseling regarding options for pregnant juveniles, including continuing or aborting the pregnancy, keeping the child, or putting it up for adoption, should be included.

Public health family planning clinics, Planned Parenthood Foundation clinics, and individual physicians are examples of community resources with which the facility can coordinate services.

Optional Recommendations

Liaisons with community clinicians should be established to facilitate programs within the facility and discharge planning.

It is advisable that a formal legal opinion on the law relating to abortion be obtained, and based on that opinion, written policy and defined procedures should be developed for the correctional facility's jurisdiction.

Because some female contraceptive methods only become effective over time, it is recommended that such methods be initiated at an appropriate time prior to discharge in keeping with the laws of the jurisdiction and wishes of the female.

Y-G-10
important

AIDS TO IMPAIRMENT

Standard

Medical and dental *orthoses* or *prostheses* and other *aids to impairment* are supplied in a timely manner when the health of the juvenile would otherwise be adversely affected, as determined by the responsible physician or dentist.

Compliance Indicators

1. Evidence that prescribed aids to impairment are received is confirmed through health record documentation.
2. Where the use of specific aids to impairment are contraindicated for security concerns, alternatives are considered so the health needs of the juvenile are met.
3. All aspects of the standard are addressed by written policy and defined procedures.

Definitions

Orthoses are specialized mechanical devices, such as braces, foot inserts, and hand splints, used to support or supplement weakened or abnormal joints or limbs.

Prostheses are artificial devices to replace missing body parts such as limbs, teeth, eyes, and heart valves.

Aids to impairment are devices such as eyeglasses, hearing aids, canes, crutches, and wheelchairs that enhance or restore physical functions.

Discussion

The standard intends that the facility provides resources to juveniles with physical impairments.

Y-G-11
important

CARE FOR THE TERMINALLY ILL

Standard

A program to address the needs of *terminally ill* juveniles includes pain management. When the responsible physician determines that care in a community setting is medically preferable, he or she recommends to the appropriate legal authority the patient's transfer or *early release*.

Compliance Indicators

1. Medical treatment and care are provided according to current community standards. Adequate and appropriate pain management is provided and documented in the health record.
2. In keeping with the requirements of the jurisdiction regarding end-of-life decisions for juvenile patients:
    a. evidence exists, through documentation in the health record, that the patient's guardian has been given sufficient and relevant information to make informed decisions, including specialty and second-opinion consultations, and that the patient is involved in the process as appropriate for his or her age and maturity.
    b. When the facility is not equipped to provide needed services, the patient is transferred to another facility, hospital, or hospice that is able to meet his or her health needs.
3. Qualified health care professionals initiate or facilitate the early release of terminally ill juveniles in a timely manner consistent with the laws of the jurisdiction.
4. All aspects of this standard are addressed in written policy and defined procedures.

Definitions

Early release refers to the release of a juvenile before the expiration of his or her sentence based on the juvenile's terminal condition. In some states, this is known as medical parole or compassionate release.

A *hospice* program delivers palliative care (medical care and support services aimed at providing comfort). Treatment is focused on symptom control and quality of life issues rather than attempting to cure conditions.

A *terminally ill* juvenile is one whose physical condition has deteriorated to the point where the prognosis is less than a year to live.

Discussion

This standard intends that the facility has a policy that addresses the needs of the terminally ill. A "good death" is generally considered to be one that takes place in a supportive environment, in dignity, without pain, and in the company of family and/or friends. The correctional system as a whole should strive for an effective program that addresses these issues for the terminally ill.

In facilities with a hospice program, enrollment is contingent on independent review, patient-centered choice, and decisions of the legal guardian consistent with the legal requirements of the jurisdiction.

Optional Recommendations

In a facility that cares for terminally ill juveniles, the child care and health staffs should receive in-service training on end-of-life issues. The impact of the dying process on the other juveniles present should be considered.

Many resources are available to correctional health staff developing hospice programs. The Volunteers of America, National Hospice and Palliative Care Organization, and the National Prison Hospice Association have guidelines for best practices of hospice care in correctional settings.

SECTION H – HEALTH RECORDS

Y-H-01
essential

HEALTH RECORD FORMAT AND CONTENTS

Standard

The method of recording entries in the health record and the format of the health record are approved by the responsible health authority.

Compliance Indicators

1. At a minimum, the health record contains these elements:
    a. identifying information (e.g., juvenile name, identification number, date of birth, sex);
    b. a problem list containing medical and mental health diagnoses and treatments as well as known allergies;
    c. receiving screening and health assessment forms;
    d. progress notes of all significant findings, diagnoses, treatments, and dispositions;
    e. clinician orders for prescribed medication and medication administration records;
    f. reports of laboratory, X-ray, and diagnostic studies;
    g. flow sheets;
    h. consent and refusal forms;
    i. release of information forms;
    j. results of specialty consultations and off-site referrals;
    k. discharge summaries of hospitalizations and other inpatient stays;
    l. special needs treatment plan, if applicable;
    m. immunization records, if applicable;
    n. place, date, and time of each clinical encounter; and
    o. signature and title of each documenter.
2. If electronic records are used, procedures address integration of health information in electronic and paper forms.
3. Where mental health or dental records are separate from medical records, a process ensures that pertinent information is shared. At a minimum, a listing of current problems and medications is common to all mental health, medical, and dental records of a juvenile.
4. All aspects of the standard are addressed by written policy and defined procedures.

Discussion

This standard intends that a health record is properly created and maintained for juveniles.

A complete health record is not necessarily established on every juvenile; however, any health intervention after the receiving screening requires the initiation of a record.

Whether clinical encounters occur in the facility or in the community, all findings are recorded in the health record. Identification of record entries may be by written signature, initials, rubber-stamped signature, or electronic signature.

The health record contains documentation of off-site consultations. The documentation from the consultant includes, at a minimum, diagnostic findings and treatment recommendations.

A unified health record comprised of all health care documents is preferable. Where the facility permits different disciplines to maintain separate health records, pertinent information is accessible and retrievable by all to facilitate continuity of care.

Optional Recommendations

The problem-oriented health record structure is recommended. Whatever health record structure is used, however, every effort should be made to establish standardization and uniformity of health record forms, order, and content.

The problem list is best kept in the front of the record.

In correctional systems with multiple facilities it is helpful to note, in the front or in a prominent place in the chart, every transfer from one facility to another so that the dates of stay at each location are clear.

Electronic health record systems should protect access and provide security of the record by the use of contemporary information technology security methods. Procedures for downtime and regular backups should be in place.

Y-H-02
essential

CONFIDENTIALITY OF HEALTH RECORDS AND INFORMATION

Standard

The confidentiality of a patient's written or electronic health record, as well as orally conveyed health information, is maintained.

Compliance Indicators

1. Health records stored in the facility are maintained under secure conditions separate from correctional records.
2. Access to health records and health information is controlled by the responsible health authority (RHA).
3. Evidence exists that health staff receive instruction in maintaining
4. confidentiality.
5. If records are transported by nonhealth staff, the records are sealed.

6. Nonhealth staff who observe or overhear a clinical encounter are instructed that they also are required to maintain confidentiality.
7. All aspects of the standard are addressed by written policy and defined procedures.

Discussion

The intent of this standard is to protect the patient's right to confidentiality of personal health information.

The principle of confidentiality protects the patient from disclosure of certain confidences entrusted to the health care professional. Thus, health records must be maintained under security and completely separate from juveniles' custody records.

At all times, including during transfers and referrals, the confidentiality of the contents of health records must be maintained.

Maintaining confidentiality of health records is to be included in the orientation program for health staff (see Y-C-09 Orientation for Health Staff) and is to be reviewed periodically. Health staff are to be reminded not to discuss patients' health information in front of child care staff or other juveniles, including those working in or near the health services area. Nonhealth staff who observe or overhear a clinical encounter are instructed that they are also required to maintain confidentiality. Evidence that staff with access to the health records have been instructed in the need for confidentiality may take several forms. These include policies and procedures, memoranda to staff, minutes of meetings, and reviews during roll call or in-services.

Optional Recommendation

The responsible health authority should maintain a current file on the rules and regulations covering the confidentiality of health records and the types of information that may and may not be shared. Local, state, or federal laws may allow certain exceptions to the obligations of health care professionals to maintain confidentiality; health staff should inform juveniles at the beginning of the health care encounter when these circumstances apply.

Y-H-03
important

ACCESS TO CUSTODY INFORMATION

Standard

Qualified health care professionals have access to information in the juvenile's custody record when the responsible health authority determines that such information may be relevant to the juvenile's health and course of treatment.

Compliance Indicator

A written policy and defined procedures specify which health staff have access to custody records, including guardian information, and under what circumstances.

Discussion

This standard intends that criminal justice information that may influence clinical decisions is available to health staff for treatment purposes.

It is not necessary or even desirable that all health staff have access to the criminal history of their patients. Yet, a juvenile's custody record may contain information relevant to the provision of health services. The juvenile's arrest and confinement record may be useful to health staff who need information regarding the juvenile's history of violence, drug and alcohol use, mental condition at the time of arrest, possession of medication, or details of the crime leading to arrest.

Y-H-04
important

MANAGEMENT OF HEALTH RECORDS

Standard

A health record is maintained to facilitate continuity of care.

Compliance Indicators

1. Evidence exists that the health record is available and used.
2. When a juvenile is transferred to another correctional facility:
   a. a copy of the current health record or a comprehensive health summary accompanies the juvenile, and
   b. unless otherwise provided by law or administrative regulation, written authorization by the juvenile or guardian (and/or parent as required by law) is required to transfer health records and information to facilities outside the correctional system's jurisdiction.
3. The jurisdiction's legal requirements regarding records retention are followed.
4. There is a system for the timely reactivation of records when requested by a treating health professional.
5. All aspects of the standard are addressed by written policy and defined procedures.

Discussion

The standard intends that the facility has a system to facilitate health record use.

Having the record available to health staff for each patient encounter enhances continuity of care, facilitates early and correct diagnosis based on review of prior symptoms and findings, and permits coordination of treatment by multiple clinicians.

This standard addresses procedures to be followed when a juvenile is transferred to a correctional facility outside the jurisdiction of the current correctional system. See Y-D-05 Hospital and Specialty Care for sharing of information when the juvenile is referred to an outside health professional, Y-E-03 Transfer Screening for procedures when the juvenile is transferred within the same correctional system, and Y-E-13 Discharge Planning for the process when the juvenile is returned to the community.

When an individual is readmitted into a correctional system, reactivation of the health record is important to facilitate continuity of care and ensure diagnostic evaluations are current.

If the paper or electronic medical record is not available during the patient encounter, health staff should so indicate on a temporary documenting form that is subsequently filed in the record.

For patients being transferred with critical or chronic health problems, the health information should be flagged to expedite an immediate referral to a clinician.

Optional Recommendations

A juvenile's health record or summary should accompany the juvenile in order to ensure continuity of care and to prevent the duplication of tests and examinations at the receiving facility.

When a juvenile is transferred to another facility in a different system, the transferring facility should provide a discharge summary or transfer form that might include the following: the medical history, the date of the last physical examination, the immunization record, a summary of medical problems, the juvenile's current health status (including oral health, mental health, and substance abuse concerns), current level of activity, current therapy (including medications), and anticipated future health care needs.

SECTION I – MEDICAL-LEGAL ISSUES

Y-I-01
essential

RESTRAINT AND SECLUSION

Standard

Clinically ordered restraint and *seclusion* are available for patients exhibiting behavior dangerous to self or others as a result of medical or mental illness. Except for monitoring their health status, the health staff does not participate in the restraint of juveniles ordered by child care staff.

Compliance Indicators

1. Juveniles are not restrained in a manner that would jeopardize their health.
2. With regard to clinically ordered restraint and seclusion (including time out):
   a. Policies and procedures specify:
      i. the types of restraints or conditions of seclusion that may be used;
      ii. when, where, how, and for how long restraints or seclusion may be used;
      iii. how proper peripheral circulation is maintained (when restraints are used); and
      iv. that proper nutrition, hydration, and toileting are provided.
   b. The least restrictive, appropriate treatment is used.
   c. In each case, use of restraint is authorized by a physician or other qualified health care professional where permitted by law.
   d. Every 15 minutes, health-trained child care staff or health staff check on any patient placed in clinically ordered restraints or seclusion. Such checks are documented.
   e. The treatment plan provides for removing patients from restraints or seclusion as soon as possible.
   f. The same types of restraints that would be appropriate for individuals treated in the community are used in the facility.
3. With regard to custody-ordered restraints:
   a. When restraints are used by child care staff for security reasons, health staff are notified immediately in order to (1) review the health record for any contraindications or accommodations required, which, if present, are immediately communicated to appropriate child care staff, and (2) initiate health monitoring, which continues at designated intervals as long as the juvenile is restrained.
   b. If the restrained juvenile has a medical or mental health condition, the physician is notified immediately so that appropriate orders can be given.
   c. When health staff note improper use of restraints that is jeopardizing the health of a juvenile, they communicate their concerns as soon as possible to appropriate child care staff.
4. All aspects of the standard are addressed by written policy and defined procedures.

Definitions

Clinically ordered restraint is a therapeutic intervention initiated by medical or mental health staff to use devices designed to safely limit a patient's mobility.

Clinically ordered seclusion is a therapeutic intervention initiated by medical or mental health staff to use rooms designed to safely limit a patient's mobility.

Discussion

This standard intends that when restraints are used for clinical or custody reasons, the juvenile is not harmed by the intervention.

When clinically ordered restraint or seclusion is used, it is employed for the shortest time possible in keeping with current community practice. Juveniles are not restrained in an unnatural position (for instance, hog-tied, facedown, spread-eagle). All staff who use restraints are trained in their proper application. Examples of typical restraint devices are fleece-lined leather, rubber or canvas hand and leg restraints, 2-point and 4-point restraints, and restraint chairs. Metal or hard plastic devices (such as handcuffs and leg shackles) are not used for clinically ordered restraint.

Generally, an order for clinical restraint or seclusion is not to exceed 1 hour, but state health code requirements, if applicable, may vary. Health monitoring consists of checks for circulation and nerve damage, airway obstruction, and psychological trauma.

Responsible health authorities (RHAs) that do not permit use of clinically ordered restraints or seclusion generally transfer patients to a local emergency room or another juvenile correctional facility equipped to offer such interventions.

This standard reflects a number of findings and assumptions:

Serious injuries and deaths, though rare, have occurred as a result of the process of applying restraints. Injuries usually occur during the restraint process but also can be the result of nerve or artery constriction. Deaths are usually the result of airway restriction (e.g., aspiration of vomitus, gagging, or covering the mouth and/or nose of the restrained person). When restraint practices are misused and result in litigation, judges have either forbidden their use or placed their use solely under the supervision of the health staff.

Many juvenile programs choose not to use fixed restraint as a behavior control measure. Programs that do use restraints have found that carefully written policies and conscientious supervision can significantly reduce restraint time and the number of restraint incidents. For this reason, it is recommended that restraints be kept in a central location, rather than on units, and their access be controlled by supervisory personnel.

When restraints are ordered by child care workers, health staff review the health record for any contraindications or accommodations required. Health staff should not be put in the position to appear to approve or to condone restraint orders by child care workers.

Optional Recommendation

In the rare instance when a juvenile would be restrained beyond 1 hour, whether ordered for clinical or custody purposes, exercising each limb for at least 10 minutes every 2 hours is recommended to prevent blood clots.

Performance Measures

1. When clinical restraint is used, juveniles receive no new injuries related to the restraint. In the event of injury, an assessment of the circumstances of the restraint focuses on whether the injury could have been prevented and whether corrective action is needed.
2. In the preceding year, and in comparison with previous years, the use of clinical restraint, expressed as ratio of the number of occurrences to the average daily population, is either stable or decreasing from the first through the last quarters of the most recent year, and overall when all years' data are reviewed. When this is not the outcome, relevant continuous quality improvement (CQI) studies are undertaken to assess root causes and take corrective action, if necessary.

Performance Measure Expectations

The expectation is that the performance measures are met 100% of the time.

The RHA decides what methods of study and documentation are to be used in internal reviews to assess compliance with these measures. All such studies and tracking methods are incorporated into the facility's CQI program.

Juveniles requiring clinical mechanical intervention are out of control and striking out; bruises, scratches, and other minor injuries, including deliberate self-mutilation, are often the result of the behavior for which the juvenile is being restrained. However the process of restraining the juvenile by itself should not result in physical injury when applied properly. Careful physical evaluation of the juvenile following restraint and documentation kept in both aggregate and individual form (measure #1) needs to be centralized for review and action if needed.

Measure #2 helps the facility to identify trends and provides an opportunity for intervention or corrective action to address issues contributing to increasing or inappropriate use of restraint. Data on the individuals in need of such intervention as well as aggregate data need to be compiled and reviewed. Explanation for increases in use of restraint with an individual or facilitywide need to be explored. Resulting study recommendations lead to corrective action.

Y-I-02
essential

EMERGENCY PSYCHOTROPIC MEDICATION

Standard

Health staff follow policies developed for the emergency use of *forced* psychotropic medications as governed by the laws applicable in the jurisdiction.

Compliance Indicators

1. The policies on forced psychotropic medication:
   a. require physician authorization prior to use, and
   b. specify when, where, and how the psychotropic medication may be forced.
2. When a physician orders psychotropic medication to be forced, he or she documents in the juvenile's record:
   a. the juvenile's condition,
   b. the threat posed,
   c. the reason for forcing the medication,
   d. other treatment modalities attempted, if any, and
   e. treatment plan goals for less restrictive treatment alternatives as soon as possible.
3. All aspects of the standard are addressed by written policy and defined procedures.

Definition

Forced medications are those given without the patient's consent.

Discussion

This standard's intent is to have a protocol for emergency situations when a juvenile is dangerous to self or others due to a medical or mental illness and when forced psychotropic medication may be used to prevent harm, based on a physician's order. The standard supports the principle that psychotropic medication may not be used simply to control behavior or as a disciplinary measure (see Y-D-02 Medication Services).

Though the right to refuse treatment is inherent in the notion of informed consent, exceptions may arise in psychiatric emergencies. State laws vary on this matter, but, as a rule, forced psychotropic medication is employed only when the juvenile is imminently dangerous to self or others due to mental disease or defect. RHAs that do not permit the use of forced psychotropic medication in an emergency generally transfer the patient immediately to a hospital emergency room for assessment and treatment.

Optional Recommendations

This standard applies to emergency situations only. For guidance in forcing psychotropic medications on a more frequent basis or as part of an ongoing treatment plan, staff are referred to case law (e.g., *Washington v. Harper*).

Y-I-03
important

FORENSIC INFORMATION

Standard

Health staff are prohibited from participating in the collection of *forensic information*.

Compliance Indicators

1. Health staff are not involved in the collection of forensic information (e.g., DNA testing) except when:
    a. complying with state laws that require blood samples from juveniles, so long as there is consent of the juvenile and health staff are not involved in any punitive action taken as a result of a juvenile's nonparticipation in the collection process,
    b. conducting body cavity searches, and blood or urine testing for alcohol or other drugs when done for medical purposes by a physician's order,
    c. conducting juvenile-specific, court-ordered laboratory tests, examinations, or radiology procedures with consent of the juvenile, and
    d. in the case of sexual assault, gathering evidence from the victim with his or her consent.
2. All aspects of the standard are addressed by written policy and defined procedures.

Definition

Forensic information is physical or psychological data collected from a juvenile that may be used against him or her in disciplinary or legal proceedings.

Discussion

The intent of this standard is to ensure that the role of the health staff is to serve the health needs of their patients. Performing psychological evaluations of juveniles for use in adversarial proceedings (e.g., court, probation, or parole hearings), conducting body cavity searches for contraband, and collecting blood or urine specimens for drug analysis are examples of ethical conflicts for health staff. Such acts undermine the credibility of these professionals with their patients and compromise health staff by asking them to participate in acts that are usually done without juveniles' consent. Where state laws and regulations require that such acts be performed by a health professional, the services of outside professionals or someone on staff who is not involved in a therapeutic relationship with the juvenile is obtained.

Alternatives to health staff participation in collecting information for forensic purposes are available in some cases. For example, in lieu of body cavity searches, a dry cell could be used; oral and buccal sampling for DNA do not require the involvement of health staff; and urine testing for drug use can be done by child care staff.

Optional Recommendation

Maintaining ethical boundaries and professional attitudes is difficult in correctional institutions. However, orientation for new hires and continuing education on potential ethical conflicts can help health staff maintain their ethical perspectives.

Body cavity searches conducted for reasons of security should be done in privacy by outside health care clinicians (as noted above) or by child care workers of the same sex as the juvenile who have been trained by a physician or other health care clinician to probe body cavities (without the use of instruments) so as to cause neither injury to tissue nor infection.

Y-I-04
important

INFORMED CONSENT AND RIGHT TO REFUSE

Standard

All examinations, treatments, and procedures are governed by *informed consent* practices for juvenile care that are applicable in the jurisdiction. A juvenile may refuse specific health evaluations and treatments in accordance with the laws in the jurisdiction.

Compliance Indicators

1. The policy and procedures specify circumstances under which risks and benefits of an intervention are explained to the patient.
2. The informed consent of next of kin, guardian, or legal custodian applies when required by law.
3. For invasive procedures or any treatment where there is risk and benefit to the patient, informed consent is documented on a written form containing the signatures of the patient, legal guardian if required, and health staff witness.
4. Any health evaluation and treatment refusal is documented and must include the following:
   a. description of the nature of the service being refused;

      b.   evidence that the juvenile has been made aware of any adverse consequences to health that may occur as a result of the refusal;

      c.   the signature of the patient; and

      d.   the signature of a health staff witness.

5.   There is evidence of involvement of the legal guardian in cases of refusal when required by the laws of the jurisdiction.

6.   In the event the patient does not sign the refusal form, it is to be noted on the form by a health staff witness.

7.   All aspects of the standard are addressed by written policy and defined procedures.

Definition

Informed consent is the agreement by a patient or guardian to a treatment, examination, or procedure after the patient or guardian receives the material facts about the nature, consequences, and risks of the proposed treatment, examination, or procedure; the alternatives to it; and the prognosis if the proposed intervention is not undertaken.

Discussion

This standard intends that juveniles use their right to make informed decisions regarding health care. Consent of the legal guardian (e.g., parents, court-appointed guardian, superintendent) as required by the jurisdiction's regulations is needed for invasive treatment or diagnostic testing. It is helpful to have the assent of the patient to the intervention; however, this is not sufficient by itself. Even when the juvenile's assent is not formally required, the juvenile's involvement in these decisions and ability to discuss them with the legal guardian and health staff is encouraged.

Medical, mental health, or dental treatment of a patient without the consent of the legal custodian can result in legal action. Some states allow juveniles to consent to treatment without consent of their legal guardian as long as they are mature enough to comprehend the consequences of their decision. Others require consent of a legal guardian until maturity, but the age of maturity varies among the states.

There are a few situations in which it is not necessary to obtain informed consent. Examples of exceptions are life-threatening conditions that require immediate medical intervention for the safety of the patient, emergency care of patients who do not have the capacity to understand the information given (see Y-I-02 Emergency Psychotropic Medication), and certain public health matters.

In facilities where upon admission a juvenile is required to give "blanket" consent for treatment by the health staff, written consents are still required for invasive procedures including surgeries, invasive diagnostic tests, and dental extractions.

Another intent of this standard is to support the ethical principle that patients have the right to refuse health interventions. A patient's refusal of care is to be an informed decision, with the consequences explained to the individual.

A blanket refusal for treatment is not permitted. By refusing treatment at a particular time, the patient does not waive the right to subsequent health care.

Juveniles may not be punished for exercising their right to refuse treatment. Even when the treatment at issue is a public health matter, there are ways to handle refusals that do not involve disciplining juveniles. For example, when the refusal pertains to a condition that poses a health risk to others, it may be appropriate to medically isolate and counsel the juvenile regarding the medical consequences of refusing treatment. Another alternative is to seek a court order forcing treatment, but only if the clinical condition warrants such an extreme measure.

In situations where the refusal may seriously jeopardize the patient's health, the individual should be brought to the medical clinic and the benefits and risks of the proposed treatment explained. The health professional can then answer any questions the patient may have. If the patient still wishes to decline the treatment, he or she should be counseled about the possible consequences of that refusal. If the patient still refuses and the condition is not life-threatening, he or she should be allowed to decline in writing.

If a juvenile refuses treatment, the responsible health authority should notify the appropriate legal guardian. Notification of the legal guardian generally is not required unless the refusal poses a substantial risk to the juvenile or the juvenile has a court-appointed guardian where notification is required. This more elaborate procedure is not generally required for refusal of routine sick call or refusal of a dose of medication. If there are no dire consequences to the refusal, the health professional may simply note in the record that the person was a no-show for sick call or refused medication.

Optional Recommendation

Laws regarding consent to treatment by juveniles, the need to involve legal guardians, and their right to refuse treatment vary from state to state. The law of the jurisdiction in which the facility is located should be reviewed by legal counsel and, based on counsel's written opinion, a policy regarding the right to refuse treatment should be developed.

Health professionals should counsel juveniles who repeatedly do not keep clinic appointments; they should continue to counsel juveniles who have refused a particular treatment when the health professional believes it to be in the patient's best interest.

Some refusals may result from system disincentives (e.g., holding sick call at a time that conflicts with other important programming) and should be addressed by exploring possible alternatives so that the conflicts are lessened or eliminated.

MEDICAL AND OTHER RESEARCH

Standard

Biomedical, behavioral, or other research using juveniles as subjects is consistent with established ethical, medical, legal, and regulatory standards for human research.

Compliance Indicators

1. Any research conducted should meet the standards for design and control, and the juvenile (or legal guardian where required by jurisdictional law) must have given informed consent.
2. When juveniles who are participants in a community-based research protocol are admitted to the facility, procedures provide for:
   a. continuation of participation, or
   b. consultation with community researchers so that withdrawal from the research protocol is done without harming the health of the juvenile.
3. All aspects of the standard are addressed by written policy and defined procedures that specify:
   a. the process for obtaining approval to conduct the research, and
   b. the steps to be taken to preserve the participant's rights.

Discussion

The standard intends to support legitimate research initiatives. Juveniles are protected from being taken advantage of due to their status.

Improvement in the quality of health care and its delivery depend on the advancement of knowledge through research. Because juveniles may be under special constraints that could affect their ability to make a truly voluntary and uncoerced decision to participate as research subjects, it is important to provide safeguards for the protection of those involved in research activities.

The Code of Federal Regulations (45 CFR 46, revised) has established special provisions that protect inmates involved in research activities. These regulations do allow, under proper conditions and with appropriate external reviews and approvals, for the participation of inmates in studies of the possible causes, effects, and processes of incarceration; studies on conditions particularly affecting inmates as a group; and research on practices, both innovative and established, that are intended and reasonably likely to improve the health and well-being of the participant.

Staff of correctional health care programs wishing to conduct research activities involving juveniles are to be knowledgeable about the pertinent federal regulations noted above.

This standard is not intended to restrict the collection of aggregate data from health record reviews (as long as confidentiality is maintained) nor to prohibit juveniles from participating in established clinical trials where there is some potential benefit to the participants(provided federal regulations are followed).

APPENDICES

The Legal Context of Correctional Health Care

From biblical times to *Bye-Bye Birdie's* "What's the matter with kids today," the treatment of errant youth has perplexed society. Historically, children, like women, were considered the property of the male head of household. While the legal notion of children or women as property has fallen away, the law nevertheless retains an inconsistent attitude toward society's children and their rights. At 18, a youth can vote for the President of the United States and don a military uniform and die in battle for country, but he or she is still regarded as lacking sufficient maturity to purchase a bottle of beer.

The age of "emancipation" or consent to make a contract or wed varies from state to state. Parents in general have the right of control over their children, but, where there are no parents or parents are unfit, guardians are appointed or children enter foster care or are made wards of the state.

Juveniles, too, have rights: to shelter, food, clothing, and education, and to be free of abuse - some of which are not bestowed on adults. These rights are enforced in some states by juveniles themselves after a certain age; in others, by adults acting for them or by the state itself, applying child abuse and neglect and truancy laws.

When juveniles disobey the criminal law, they may find themselves in custody or placement in some form of institutional setting. While historically juvenile offenders were separated by law from adult convicts,[1] many states now allow treatment of certain juvenile offenders as adults. Some jurisdictions place older juveniles who seriously offend in institutions designed for adults (Glick & Sturgeon, 1998),[2] while others confine juveniles in facilities built especially for them. Although the nature of institutionalization may vary from state to state (or even within a state), all juveniles in custody have the right to health care.

Juveniles' Right to Health Care in Custody

A parent's failure to provide a child with proper health care can result in a finding of neglect, and, in extreme cases, removal of the child from that home. When a child is arrested, found to be delinquent, and incarcerated by the government, this obligation for health care falls upon the government as a matter of constitutional law, enforceable under the U.S. Constitution's due process clauses of the Fifth Amendment (for juveniles in federal custody) and of the 14th Amendment (for juveniles in state and local custody). Where the incarceration of the juvenile is for the conviction of a crime, the Constitution's Eighth Amendment (which prohibits "cruel and unusual punishment") also establishes a federal right to medical care where failure to provide it amounts to deliberate indifference to serious medical needs, a standard established by the U.S. Supreme Court in the landmark decision *Estelle v. Gamble*.[3]

In the hundreds of published cases following *Estelle*, three basic rights have emerged: the right to access to care, the right to care that is ordered, and the right to a professional medical judgment. Although there has been some fine-tuning, the legal landscape has remained largely unchanged for more than 25 years.

To provide for constitutional care and to protect themselves from litigation, correctional administrators must adopt procedures to protect juveniles' basic rights, including a functioning sick-call system that uses properly trained health care staff, a means of addressing medical emergencies, a priority system so that those most in need of care receive it first, the development and maintenance of adequate medical records, liaison with outside resources for specialist and hospital care when needed, a system for staff development and training, and an ongoing effort at quality control. Custodial executives and their chief medical officers must develop policies and procedures for meeting the special needs of disabled and mentally ill juveniles, as well as those with HIV infection and AIDS, and to preserve the confidentiality of medical information.

Because litigation is so expensive, all efforts should be made to achieve voluntary compliance with national standards of care and to gain accreditation. Facilities that meet community standards of care are much less likely to face class action or even individual lawsuits.

The Constitutional Standard

The standard of liability under the Constitution is relatively narrow. The Constitution does not render prison officials or staff liable in federal cases for malpractice or accidents, nor does it resolve professional disputes about the best choice of treatment (*Ramsey v. Ciccone*).[4] It does require, however, that sufficient resources be made available to protect the three basic rights.

While the constitutional standard does not require that an express intent to inflict pain be shown (*Wilson v. Seiter*),[5] it does include an inquiry into the defendant's state of mind. A violation requires a "subjective" showing of "deliberate indifference." It is not enough that the defendant should have known or understood the danger to the inmate. The defendant must know of and disregard a substantial risk (*Farmer v. Brennan*).[6] Such knowledge, however, can be inferred from the surrounding facts where the failure to respond to a clear risk is reckless.

The Right to Access to Care
The right to access to care is fundamental: When access is denied or delayed, the health staff does not know which patients need immediate attention and which patients need care that can wait. Indeed, "[a] well-monitored and well-run access system is the best way to protect prisoners from unnecessary harm and suffering and, concomitantly, to protect prison officials from liability for denying access to needed medical care" (Winner, 1981).[7]

The right to access to care includes access to both emergency and routine care. All institutions, of whatever size, must have the capacity to cope with emergencies and to provide for sick call. Access to specialists and to inpatient hospital treatment, where warranted by the patient's condition, are also guaranteed by the Constitution.

The Right to Care That Is Ordered
Generally, courts assume that care would not have been ordered if it were not needed. Thus, once a health care professional orders treatment for a serious condition, the courts will protect, as a matter of constitutional law, the patient's right to receive that treatment without undue delay. The easiest way for an institution to lose a lawsuit is to fail to provide inmate patients with the care that its own medical staff has ordered.

The Right to a Professional Medical Judgment
In general, the courts will not determine which of two equally efficacious treatment modalities should be chosen. The adjudication of constitutional claims is not the business of "second-guessing" health care professionals. Rather, the courts seek to:

> ...ensure that decisions concerning the nature and timing of medical care are made by medical personnel, using equipment designed for medical use, in locations conducive

to medical functions, and for reasons that are purely medical.

Neisser, 1977[8]

By ensuring that professional judgment is actually exercised, however, the federal courts not only have protected the sphere of discretion surrounding medical practitioners' treatment and diagnostic decisions, but also have often enhanced it. At issue in a typical injunctive case are such matters as staffing, physical facilities, transportation, and sick call and follow-up procedures. When a court orders relief in these areas, it is assuring that the raw materials from which responsible professional judgment is formed and carried out are available to practitioners.

Serious Medical Needs

The Constitution requires that correctional officials provide medical care only for serious medical needs. Generally, a medical need is "serious" if it "has been diagnosed by a physician as mandating treatment or...is so obvious that even a lay person would easily recognize the necessity for a doctor's attention" (*Duran v. Anaya; Ramos v. Lamm*).[9] Conditions are also considered to be serious if they "cause pain, discomfort, or threat to good health" (*Dean v. Coughlin*).[10] A condition need not be life-threatening to be deemed serious, and many treatment plans that are labeled "elective" nevertheless are deemed serious within the meaning of *Estelle v. Gamble*.

In general, courts consider three factors in determining whether correctional officials are being deliberately indifferent to serious medical needs: (1) the amenability of the patient's condition to treatment, (2) the consequences to the patient if treatment does not occur, and (3) the likelihood of a favorable outcome. Within this mix, the court may also consider the length of the patient's anticipated incarceration (Rold, 1997).[11]

The Constitutional Class Action Challenge

Class action challenges to correctional health care delivery are put together in two ways, either of which is independently sufficient (*Todaro v. Ward*).[12] First, numerous examples of individual cases of deliberate indifference closely related in time can establish a pattern of unconstitutional care. Alternatively, evidence of systemic deficiencies in staffing, facilities, record keeping, supervision, and procedures can show that unnecessary suffering is inevitable unless the deficiencies are remedied (*Bishop v. Stoneman*).[13] Juvenile institutions are not immune from class action lawsuits, including investigation and litigation by civil rights groups or the U.S. Department of Justice (Lewis and Consoulin, 2004).[14]

The best preventive medicine against a successful class action challenge is adequate funding. A recent study found that health care costs for incarcerated juveniles exceeded the average cost for adult inmates and that nearly 75% of all health care costs for juveniles were for mental health services (Tennyson, 2003).[15] An adequate system also needs sound procedures, adherence to standards, staff training, and quality control.

Components of a Constitutional System

A constitutional system of health care delivery combines a number of critical elements, each of which serves to reinforce the others. Among these are the following:

A Communications and Sick-call System

Prisoners must be permitted to communicate their emergency and routine health care needs to the medical staff, and sick call must be available to all inmates regardless of security classification (*Hoptowit v. Ray*).[16] Adequate sick call requires a professional evaluation by trained personnel. Uniform or lay staff may convey sick-call requests, but they cannot be allowed to decide which prisoners will receive medical attention (*Boswell v. Sherburne County; Kelley v. McGinnis; Mitchell v. Aluisi*).[17]

A Priority System

A system with scarce resources must set priorities calculated to relieve pain and to restore function in accordance with the seriousness of the patients' conditions. A priority system for care is not only more equitable for the patients (*see* Conte, 1983),[18] but also is one that parallels the concerns of the courts in evaluating the constitutional sufficiency of systems under review.

The courts recognize that no correctional clinic can provide complete state-of-the-art health care or the full range of available health services to unincarcerated persons, but, where such issues are resolved in accordance with a reasonable priority system, courts are likely to defer to it in determining what care is appropriate.

Personnel

Most cases in which courts have found constitutional violations of inmates' rights to health care were fostered by the exigencies of an overburdened staff coping with too few resources, and the courts will impose specific requirements when circumstances warrant. A large institution may be required to have full-time health professionals, including physicians, on site with 24-hour coverage (*Ramos v. Lamm*).[19] Even the smallest county jails, however, must have a means (such as an on-call system and officers trained in first aid) to deal with medical emergencies when no health care staff is present (*Green v. Carlson*).[20] The National Commission on Correctional Health Care offers certification as a correctional health professional to health care employees in corrections and others, based on credentials, experience, and a written examination.

Contracting Services

Many facilities have turned to contractual providers in their search for personnel and cost containment. Some state systems have contracted out their entire health care delivery system. The use of independent contractors, however, does not relieve the institution (or the contractors) of legal responsibility for health care (*West v. Atkins*).[21]

Medical Records

Maintenance of adequate medical records is "a necessity" (*Johnson-El v. Schoemehl*),[22] and numerous courts have condemned the failure to maintain an organized and complete system of health care records. At a minimum, records should be kept separately for each patient and include a medical history and problem list, notations of patient complaints, treatment progress notes, and laboratory, x-ray, and specialist findings. Not only do proper medical records promote continuity of care and protect the health and safety of the inmate population, but they also provide correctional administrators with evidence of the course of treatment when individual inmates sue them asserting that care was not provided (Kay, 1991).[23]

"Outside" Care

No correctional facility can provide complete medical care within its confines. If an inmate requires a specialist evaluation, a sophisticated diagnostic test, or inpatient care that is not available in the correctional system, the failure to provide it may constitute deliberate indifference. In such cases, security and administrative considerations concerning transportation and cost must yield to medical determinations where a particular patient is in need of prompt treatment (*United States v. State of Michigan; Ancata v. Prison Health Services*).[24]

Facilities and Resources
Space and supplies must be adequate to meet the health care needs of the institutional population (*Langley v. Coughlin*).[25] Dangerous or unsanitary physical conditions, inadequate or defective space or equipment, or unavailability of medications or other items such as eyeglasses, dentures, braces, prostheses, or special diets can all lead to violations of the Constitution.

Quality Assurance, Accreditation, and Compliance With Standards
Quality assurance has been defined as "[a] process of ongoing monitoring and evaluation to assess the adequacy and appropriateness of the care provided and to institute corrective action as needed" (Anno, 2001).[26] It is an essential aspect of any well-run system, and, in its absence, courts have often imposed external audits or appointed monitors over health care services as part of a remedy for constitutional violations and to ensure compliance with court orders (*see* Byland, 1983; *Lightfoot v. Walker*).[27]

Several national bodies offer accreditation to correctional facilities. Unlike standards of other accrediting bodies, however, the standards of the National Commission on Correctional Health Care address only health care as delivered in correctional facilities.[28]

Much of the impetus for compliance with national standards and the move toward accreditation has come from litigation. Compliance with national standards and accreditation, while not dispositive on the outcome of litigation,[29] is frequently regarded favorably by the courts. For a facility faced with court allegations of unconstitutional care, voluntary compliance with national standards and movement toward accreditation are not only hedges against liability but also sound investments in quality of care.

Special Needs and Populations

Reflecting society, juvenile institutions have many inmates who have special health care needs. Medical and mental health services must adjust to provide the individualized care the patients require.

Disabled Inmates
That fact that unusual accommodations may be necessary, in light of their special needs, to accomplish the provision of minimal conditions of incarceration does not absolve correctional officials of their duty toward handicapped inmates (*Ruiz v. Estelle*).[30] Thus, inmates who cannot walk are entitled to wheelchairs or necessary prostheses and braces, and patients with impaired hearing or vision are entitled to assistance (*Johnson v. Hardin County, Ky; Cummings v. Roberts*).[31]

Mental Health Care
Denial of adequate mental health care for juveniles with serious mental health needs may be unconstitutional under the same "deliberate indifference" standard applied to other medical needs. A mental health need is "serious" if it "has caused significant disruption in an inmate's everyday life and...prevents his functioning in the general population without disturbing or endangering others or himself" (*Tillery v. Owens*).[32]

Institutions must provide mental health screening intake to identify serious problems, including potential suicides (*Balla v. Idaho State Board of Corrections*)[33], treatment for serious conditions by mental health professionals (*Smith v. Jenkins*)[34], and training of officers to deal with mentally ill inmates (*Langley v. Coughlin*).[35] Additionally, there must be some means of separating severely mentally ill inmates from the mentally healthy. Mixing mentally ill inmates with those who are not mentally ill may violate the rights of both groups. Finally, failure to provide treatment for mentally retarded inmates may also violate the Constitution, if regression occurs (*see* Ellis & Luckasson, 1985; NCCHC, 2003).[36]

In *Washington v. Harper*,[37] the Supreme Court ruled that inmates have a "significant liberty interest" in avoiding the unwanted administration of antipsychotic drugs. The court approved such use only where certain procedural protections were available.

Except in cases of short transfers for evaluation purposes, inmates are also entitled to notice and a hearing before being committed to a mental hospital because the stigmatizing consequences of a psychiatric commitment and the possible involuntary subjection to psychiatric treatment constitute a deprivation of liberty requiring due process (*Vitek v. Jones*).[38] Psychiatric treatment may not be imposed for disciplinary purposes (*Knecht v. Gillman*),[39] and use of seclusion and restraint must be based on professional judgment reasonably related to its purpose (*Wells v. Franzen*).[40]

Pregnancy and Abortion

The number of pregnant juveniles who are incarcerated is substantial. Treatment for the complications of pregnancy (or to avoid them) constitutes a serious health care need within the meaning of the Constitution (*Boswell v. Sherburne County*).[41] The termination of an unwanted pregnancy is also considered a serious medical need, and the denial of an abortion constitutes deliberate indifference, regardless of the juvenile's ability to pay (*Monmouth County Correctional Institutional Inmates v. Lanzaro*).[42]

AIDS and HIV Infection

In general, claims of inadequate medical care for AIDS and HIV infection are evaluated under the same deliberate indifference standard as other medical care claims. Juvenile facilities must have the means to diagnose, treat, and educate their youth regarding the diseases associated with HIV and AIDS.

Legal-Ethical Considerations

Correctional facilities impose unusual constrictions on the delivery of medical services. They can be particularly difficult to navigate in juvenile facilities.

The Provider-Patient Relationship

The provider-patient relationship in corrections is imposed by the state on both the inmate and the health care provider. The inmate cannot go elsewhere, and the provider cannot fire the patient.

Confidentiality

Inmates have a constitutional right to privacy in their medical diagnoses and other health care records and information (*Woods v. White; Doe v. Coughlin*).[43] That right is not violated by the reporting of medical findings in the ordinary course of facility medical care operations or probably even to facility executives with a reason to know, but the "[c]asual, unjustified dissemination of confidential medical information to nonmedical staff and other prisoners" is unconstitutional (*Woods v. White*).[44]

In *Powell v. Schriver*,[45] the court ruled that an HIV-positive inmate had a constitutionally protected right to privacy in his or her HIV status. Relying on its earlier decision in *Doe v. City of New York*,[46] the court ruled that "the gratuitous disclosure of an inmate's confidential medical information as humor or gossip...is not reasonably related to a legitimate penological interest."

In contrast, there are occasions when a provider may have not only a prerogative but also a duty to report or disclose confidential medical information to third parties. If a concrete risk to an identifiable person is revealed and "disclosure is essential to avert danger," the revelation of a patient's private communication may be essential to prevent peril to innocent persons. In such cases, disclosure must be done "discreetly" and in a way that preserves the privacy of the patient "to the fullest extent compatible with the prevention of the threatened danger" (*Tarasoff v. Regents of the University of California*).[47]

The Right to Refuse Treatment

A mentally competent adult has a constitutional right to refuse medical treatment, including the direction that life-saving or other extraordinary measures be withdrawn in terminal cases (*Cruzan v. Missouri Department of Health*).[48] As Judge Cardozo stated almost 80 years ago: "Every human being of adult years and sound mind has a right to determine what shall be done with his own body" (*Schloendorff v. Society of New York Hospitals*).[49] This right extends to the incarcerated, as well (*White v. Napoleon*).[50]

The right has never been regarded as absolute, however (*see Comm'n of Correction v. Myers*),[51] and it may be overridden if there are strong public health reasons to administer treatment, as when the Supreme Court upheld mandatory smallpox vaccination in 1905, despite the patient's religious objections (*Jacobson v. Massachusetts*).[52] Inmates have been required, for example, to submit to blood and tuberculosis tests and to diphtheria and tetanus injections (*Thompson v. City of Los Angeles; Zaire v. Dalsheim; Ballard v. Woodard*).[53]

The right to refuse is based on the concept of informed consent. As one court stated:

> A prisoner's right to refuse treatment is useless without knowledge of the proposed treatment. Prisoners have a right to such information as is reasonably necessary to make an informed decision to accept or reject proposed treatment, as well as a reasonable explanation of the viable alternative treatments that can be made available in a prison setting.
>
> *White v. Napoleon*[54]

In many states, juveniles may lack legal capacity to consent (or to refuse) medical procedures, and parental consent may be required. In other states, the warden or state may assume this role *in loco parentis* upon the juvenile's conviction. In still other places, a judge's approval must be obtained. In all cases involving juveniles, a second inquiry under local law must occur as to whether the consent (or refusal) obtained from the patient is legally authorized in the jurisdiction where the juvenile is confined.

There are "reason[s] to be leery of refusals of care in prisons" (Anno, 2001),[55] particularly with juveniles. Care must be taken in corrections to determine if a refusal of care is genuine.

Juveniles as Subjects in Behavioral and Biomedical Research

Like their adult counterparts, juveniles may seek to participate in medical research, and society may benefit from the findings of such research. Because of concern about juveniles in general and incarcerated subjects in particular, there are strict guidelines and protections limiting and regulating such research under federal and state law. Institutional review boards approving and monitoring research involving institutionalized juveniles must meet two separate subparts of the federal regulations governing human research, since the subjects are protected both as prisoners (Subpart C)[56] and as juveniles (Subpart D).[57] The National Commission on Correctional Health Care also has a standard (Y-I-05) applicable to research using incarcerated juveniles.

Conclusion

"No serious student of American correctional history can deny that litigation has provided the impetus for reform of medical practice in prisons and jails" (Nathan, 1985).[58] Yet, as resources become increasingly scarce, government officials are constantly faced with doing more with less, and the expense of litigation should not absorb funds that are available to upgrade delivery of services. Voluntary adoption of community standards and accreditation are a less tortuous road to reform and, in the long run, are likely to be more successful and less divisive.

Assuring constitutional health care to juveniles is a daunting task. The courts remain involved in assuring that constitutional minima are provided. With juveniles, as with adults, the protection of basic rights to access to care, to care that is ordered, and to professional judgment can be achieved without litigation where correctional administrators and health care professionals work together from within to promote excellence and strive continually to upgrade the quality of the care that is delivered.

Contribution

This appendix originally appeared in the 2004 edition of *Standards for Health Services in Juvenile Detention and Confinement Facilities*. It is reprinted here with permission of the author, William J. Rold, JD, CCHP-A.

Endnotes

1. See Juvenile Justice and Delinquency Prevention Act, 42 U.S.C. §§ 5633(a)(12)-(14), and Youth Corrections Act, 18 U.S.C. §§ 5005-5026.

2. See Glick and Sturgeon, *No Time to Play: Youthful Offenders in Adult Correctional Systems*, American Correctional Association (1998).

3. *Estelle v. Gamble*, 429 U.S. 97, 97 S.Ct. 285 (1976).

4. *Ramsey v. Ciccone*, 305 F.Supp. 600 (W.D.Mo. 1970). This important distinction survives today and must be kept in mind: One may escape constitutional liability and yet be responsible for damages under state law for simple negligence.

5. *Wilson v. Seiter*, 501 U.S. 294, 111 S.Ct. 2321 (1991).

6. *Farmer v. Brennan*, 511 U.S. 825, 114 S.Ct. 1970 (1994).

7. Winner, "An Introduction to the Constitutional Law of Prison Medical Care," 1 *J. of Prison Health* 67 (1981).

8. Neisser, "Is There a Doctor in the Joint? The Search for Constitutional Standards for Prison Health Care," 63 *Va. L. Rev.* 921 (1977).

9. *Duran v. Anaya*, 642 F.Supp. 510, 524 (D.N.M. 1986); *Ramos v. Lamm*, 639 F.2d 559, 575 (10th Cir. 1980).

10. *Dean v. Coughlin*, 623 F.Supp. 392 (S.D.N.Y. 1985).

11. Rold, "An Examination of Medical Necessity and the Law," 11 *CorrectCare* (Winter 1997).

12. *Todaro v. Ward*, 431 F.Supp. 1129 (S.D.N.Y.), *aff'd*, 565 F.2d 48 (2d Cir. 1977).

13. *Bishop v. Stoneman*, 508 F.2d 1224 (2d Cir. 1974).

14. For a description of class action litigation involving Louisiana's juvenile facilities, which included medical, dental, and mental health services and resulted in a settlement, see Lewis and Consoulin, "Navigating Your Way Through Class-Action Lawsuits," *Corrections Today* (February 2004) pp. 28-31.

15. Tennyson, "The High Cost of Health Care Within the Juvenile Justice System," 10 *J. of Correctional Health Care* 89-108 (Spring 2003).

16. *Hoptowit v. Ray*, 682 F.2d 1237 (9th Cir. 1982).

17. *Boswell v. Sherburne County*, 849 F.2d 1117 (10th Cir. 1988); *Kelley v. McGinnis*, 899 F.2d 612 (7th Cir. 1990); *Mitchell v. Aluisi*, 872 F.2d 577 (4th Cir. 1989).

18. Conte, "Dental Treatment for Incarcerated Individuals: For Whom? How Much?" 3 *J. of Prison and Jail Health* 25 (1983).

19. *Ramos v. Lamm*, 639 F.2d 559 (10th Cir. 1980).

20. *Green v. Carlson*, 581 F.2d 669 (2d Cir. 1978), *aff'd*, 446 U.S.14 (1980).

21. *West v. Atkins*, 487 U.S. 42, 108 S.Ct. 2250 (1988).

22. *Johnson-El v. Schoemehl*, 878 F.2d 1043 (8th Cir. 1989).

23. Kay, *The Constitutional Dimensions of an Inmate's Right to Health Care*, National Commission on Correctional Health Care (1991).

24. *United States v. State of Michigan*, 680 F.Supp. 928 (W.D. Mich. 1987); *Ancata v. Prison Health Services*, 769 F.2d. 700 (11th Cir. 1985).

25. *Langley v. Coughlin*, 888 F.2d 252 (2d Cir. 1989).

26. Anno, *Correctional Health Care: Guidelines for the Management of an Adequate Delivery System*, U.S. Dept. of Justice, National Institute of Corrections (2001) p. 327.

27. Byland, "Dental Care in Prisons: Quality Assurance of Dental Programs," address to Second World Congress on Prison Health Care, Ottawa (1983); *Lightfoot v. Walker*, 486 F.Supp. 504 (S.D. Ill. 1980).

28. As of May 1999, NCCHC had accredited 226 jails, 212 prisons, and 36 juvenile facilities. "NCCHC Surveyors' World" (May 1999).

29. Although the Supreme Court referred to United Nations standards in *Estelle v. Gamble*, 429 U.S. 97, 103 n.8, 97 S.Ct. 285, 290 n.8 (1976), it did not base its decision on this ground. Later, in *Rhodes v. Chapman*, 452 U.S. 337, 343, 101 S.Ct. 2392, 2397 (1981), the Court upheld double-celling at the Southern Ohio Correctional Facility at Lucasville, even though the space per inmate was less than the 60-80 square feet specified in standards of the American Correctional Association.

30. *Ruiz v. Estelle*, 503 F.Supp. 1265 (S.D. Tex. 1980), *aff'd in part and rev'd in part*, 679 F.2d 1115 (5th Cir. 1982).

31. *Johnson v. Hardin County, Ky.*, 908 F.2d 1280 (6th Cir. 1990); *Cummings v. Roberts*, 628 F.2d 1065 (8th Cir. 1980).

32. *Tillery v. Owens*, 719 F.Supp. 1256 (W.D.Pa. 1989), *aff'd*, 907 F.2d 418 (3d Cir. 1990).

33. *Balla v. Idaho State Board of Corrections*, 595 F.Supp. 1558 (D. Idaho 1984).

34. *Smith v. Jenkins*, 919 F.2d 90 (8th Cir. 1990).

35. *Langley v. Coughlin*, 888 F.2d 252 (2d Cir. 1989).

36. Ellis & Luckasson, "Mentally Retarded Criminal Defendants," 53 Geo. Wash. L. Rev. 414 (1985); *Correctional Mental Health Care: Standards & Guidelines for Delivering Services*, National Commission on Correctional Health Care (Chicago, 2003).

37. *Washington v. Harper*, 494 U.S. 210, 110 S.Ct. 1028 (1989).

38. *Vitek v. Jones*, 445 U.S. 480, 100 S.Ct. 1254 (1980).

39. *Knecht v. Gillman*, 488 F.2d 1136 (8th Cir. 1973).

40. *Wells v. Franzen*, 777 F.2d 1258, 1264-65 (7th Cir. 1985).

41. *Boswell v. Sherburne County*, 849 F.2d 1117 (10th Cir. 1988).

42. *Monmouth County Correction Institutional Inmates v. Lanzaro*, 834 F.2d 326 (3d Cir. 1987).

43. *Woods v. White*, 689 F.Supp. 874 (W.D. Wisc. 1988); *Doe v. Coughlin*, 697 F.Supp. 1234 (N.D.N.Y. 1988).

44. *Woods v. White*, 689 F.Supp. 874 (W.D. Wisc. 1988).

45. *Powell v. Schriver*, 1999 WL 223434 (2d Cir. 1999).

46. *Doe v. City of New York*, 15 F.3d 264 (2d Cir. 1994).

47. *Tarasoff v. Regents of the University of California*, 551 P.2d 334 (Cal. 1976).

48. *Cruzan v. Missouri Department of Health*, 497 U.S.261, 110 S.Ct. 2841 (1990).

49. *Schloendorff v. Society of New York Hospitals*, 211 N.Y. 125 (1914).

50. *White v. Napoleon*, 897 F.2d 103 (3d Cir. 1990).

51. *Commission of Correction v. Myers*, 399 N.E.2d 452 (Mass. 1979).

52. *Jacobson v. Massachusetts*, 197 U.S. 11 (1905).

53. *Thompson v. City of Los Angeles*, 885 F.2d 1439 (9th Cir. 1989); *Zaire v. Dalsheim*, 698 F.Supp. 57 (S.D.N.Y. 1988); *Zaire v. Dalsheim*, 698 F.Supp. 57 (S.D.N.Y. 1988).

54. *White v. Napoleon*, 897 F.2d 103 (3d Cir. 1990).

55. Anno, *Correctional Health Care: Guidelines for the Management of an Adequate Delivery System*, U.S. Dept. of Justice, National Institute of Corrections (2001) p. 56.

56. 45 C.F.R., Part 46, Subpart C.

57. 45 C.F.R., Part 46, Subpart D.

58. Nathan, "Guest Editorial," 5 *J. of Prison Health* 1 (1985).

Compliance Indicators and Performance Measures

Compliance Indicators

The NCCHC accreditation process has a unique educational component whereby NCCHC surveyors and staff provide guidance to health care providers and administrators, helping them to understand how to use the standards to develop an effective and efficient system of health care delivery. The standards, however, are intended for all correctional administrators and health staff, whether or not they work at an accredited facility. To help all users of the standards understand how compliance is measured, this manual features the compliance indicators that accreditation surveyors use when conducting surveys. These indicators will enable users to assess their facility's compliance with each standard.

Performance Measures

Having an effective and efficient health care delivery system does not assure that appropriate health care is provided. To help users assess the adequacy of patient care, selected standards also feature performance measures. These measures are a practical way to assess the degree to which the intent of these standards - good patient care - is being met.

The need to measure patient care via a continuous quality improvement (CQI) program remains an essential component of the Juvenile Standards. This edition provides simple, useful tests to measure the effectiveness of health services.

Performance measures are provided for the following standards:

Y-E-02   Receiving Screening,
Y-E-04   Health Assessment,
Y-E-08   Emergency Services,
Y-E-09   Segregated Juveniles,
Y-G-02   Patients With Special Health Needs,
Y-G-05   Suicide Prevention Program, and
Y-I-01   Restraint and Seclusion.

Those seeking NCCHC accreditation should note that these are internal tools; achieving the stated goal of the performance measure is not required. The performance measures are intended to be used in conjunction with the standard's compliance indicators and to supplement the facility's CQI efforts.

For example, for essential standard Y-E-04 Health Assessment, one measurable outcome required for compliance is that all youth receive a complete health assessment within 7 days of admission (compliance indicator #1). From a clinical standpoint, however, meeting a time requirement does not consider how effective the assessment was in identifying health problems nor whether identified health problems were appropriately addressed.

The performance measures in this manual go beyond a simple "count and report" approach to quality improvement. Such exercises are of dubious value and, indeed, may be counterproductive for many reasons, an important one being the waste of valuable staff time. Instead, the approach taken is to highlight several standards where performance measures, in conjunction with compliance indicators, can be used as a proxy for reasonably assessing the effectiveness of the care provided. The performance measures enable in-depth evaluation of one or more aspects of the selected standard, as well as assessment of compliance with its intent.

Continuous Quality Improvement

Why Bother?

It is reasonable to ask, "Why bother making the effort to implement a quality improvement program in a correctional setting?" Correctional professionals working in facilities that have implemented such programs describe at least four major benefits that they have experienced:

1. Enhanced correctional health staff cooperation. When correctional and health care staff participate jointly in quality improvement training and teams, cooperative working relationships flourish. Working side-by-side toward mutually agreed-on goals moves staff beyond traditional jurisdictional conflicts that plague prison work.[3]

2. Decreased tensions or friction with inmates. Institutions that have well-run services are easier to manage. Although bank robber Willie Sutton is oft quoted in medicine for his "go where the money is" wisdom, his perhaps more important insight was his statement that every prison riot is due, in part, to poor medical care.[4] Good medical services are important, but good meals and responsive legal services and case management all result in fewer problems with inmates at well-run facilities.

3. Increased staff satisfaction. When workers are able to participate in redesigning the programs in which they work, they tend to experience greater job satisfaction.[5] This both enhances the ability to recruit new staff as well as increases staff retention. Because few physicians or nurses graduate from professional school with strong a priori desires to work in a correctional setting, attracting and retaining competent, talented, dedicated staff is a prerequisite for high quality and a result of meaningful quality improvement programs.

4. Cost-effectiveness. Quality improvement programs throughout the country have been able to demonstrate savings by improving both the processes and outcomes of care. By improving facility or patient compliance with medication regimens, there is likely to be less morbidity, less use of outside emergency departments, and less use of outside hospitals. By attending to needlessly complex or flawed processes, one can uncover an enormous amount of waste (often as much as 40% to 50% of expenditures in health facilities) and uproot it.[6,7]

Many working in prisons are highly motivated to improve quality but are seeking a better theoretical and practical framework to guide their efforts. In this chapter, we propose some ideas and offer some suggestions for projects. We begin with a brief overview of the history of formal efforts to improve the quality of health services. We offer a number of powerful change concepts and lessons derived from basic industrial quality improvement principles as well as from our personal experiences and efforts. We then describe the unique problems and obstacles complicating efforts to improve quality in correctional settings. Finally, we offer suggestions on how to organize and implement a quality improvement program, and we provide examples of specific quality improvement problems that have been addressed successfully.

How to Organize a Quality Improvement Program

The two fundamental elements of a CQI program are management commitment and staff participation. As elementary and self-evident as this may seem, with rare exceptions, these two prerequisites are either totally lacking or fulfilled only through token involvement. Genuine commitment to these two foundations is best structurally codified in the form of a management quality council and multidisciplinary teams.[20]

The quality council is an organizational structure that is responsible for developing the annual quality improvement plan and overseeing and evaluating its implementation and effectiveness. The warden, or equivalent executive leader, along with other top leaders from the health care program should sit on the quality council.[34] These are busy people, easily distracted by many other important competing demands on their time. However, unless there is active involvement and investment of time by such senior staff, it is unlikely that the quality improvement program will do more than raise expectations and frustrations and waste considerable organizational energies for minimal returns.

The council should meet on a regular basis (usually once monthly). Its oversight role includes ensuring that the quality improvement program:

1. Is in sync with the organizational mission and priorities by empowering and coordinating process teams in key strategic areas
2. Is comprehensive in its scope, which means that it broadly addresses each of the key services (i.e., sick call, reception and transfer processes, infirmary services, dental services, medication services, chronic illness services, outside referral and specialty services, ancillary services, mental health services, and outside hospitalization)
3. Is adequately supported in terms of staff time and resources
4. Is data driven, continuously evaluated for progress, and relentlessly striving for further improvement

To effectively implement a quality improvement program, one must begin by training leadership staff, including both health care and correctional staff, in quality improvement principles and techniques. Some of this training may be done in lectures, seminars, or workshops. Other training can be done in a just-in-time manner when there is a need to learn how to engage a particular problem.

If the quality council is the backbone of an institution's quality efforts, then multidisciplinary teams are the real guts of the program.[20] It is in teams that problems are broken down and digested, and it is in teams that the absorbing task of understanding how work processes are actually carried out and how they can be improved occurs. Each team should have a trained leader and should consist of representative staff who provide services in a given area. Thus, physicians, nurses, clerks, and other staff who perform sick call or who provide urgent care should participate in those respective teams. One goal of the program might be that every health care staff member participates in at least one quality improvement team during the course of the year.

Through their intimate knowledge of the work processes, team members can share their understanding of how the patient is supposed to move, for example, through the system for a sick call encounter. This understanding entails elaboration of how "on paper" the system is supposed to work, how in practice it actually occurs, and where it stumbles. Many administrators consider the making and enforcing of rules as the sine qua non for well-run operations. CQI teaches us that there are much greater quality gains possible from understanding why glitches occur and how these variations from the ideal relate to the fundamental ways the processes are designed.[16] By rigidly imposing prescriptive rules to correct problems, administrators not only succumb to blinders resulting from their limited views of the process, but also frustrate or squash the creative energies and opportunities for diminishing barriers across disciplines (discussed previously).

Summary

What we learn from quality improvement is that, if we're just doing our jobs, then we're not doing our jobs. Just working in the same old ways is no longer sufficient. In industry, it means that we will have no job if our firm can't continuously improve so that it can keep pace with the competition. In prisons, ... well, what does it mean? If prisons are a growth industry, and it looks like they'll always be around, will there be no competition to drive us out of business?

What it means for those of us working with prisoners is that doing our jobs, or even doing our jobs better, is not enough. Privatization issues notwithstanding,[33] we have a special responsibility to the prisoners and to the larger society to draw the circles even wider. Few of us could justify our work if we were guards or doctors in a concentration camp, even an efficient, well-run camp. Continuous quality improvement's implied dissatisfaction with the status quo means that we have to more broadly challenge the status quo that we observe in prisons.[5,18]

Making the commitment to give quality care to each prisoner and to respect the human dignity of each inmate, along with our faith in the potential of the employees, is crucial to challenging the unfair, violence-prone, and vengeful forces that are filling our jails and prisons. Shining a light on these dark problems, linking hands with others who have a basic faith in human nature and who believe in humane care, and striving to improve individuals' conditions and their lives should, in the end, be what high-quality caring means for this population.

Contribution

This appendix is excerpted from a chapter in *Clinical Practice in Correctional Medicine* (Michael Puisis, DO, editor), "Challenges of Improving Quality in the Correctional Setting," pp. 491-502, © 2008 Elsevier.

References

3. Squires N: Promoting health in prisons. BMJ 313:1161, 1996.

4. Reynolds Q: I, Willie Sutton. Paperback Library, 1953.

5. Goldfield N and Schiff G: Continuous quality improvement at the cross-roads: Contradictions and challenges. Managed Care Q 5:10-18, 1997.

6. Berwick DM: Continuous improvement as an ideal in health care. N Engl J Med 320:53-56, 1989.

7. Berwick DM: A primer on leading the improvement of systems. BMJ 312:619-622, 1996.

16. Walton M: The Deming Management Method. New York: Perigee, 1986.

18. Schiff GD and Goldfield NI: Deming meets Braverman: Toward a progressive analysis of the continuous quality improvement paradigm. Int J Health Serv 24:655-673, 1994.

20. Scholtes PR, Joiner BL, Braswell B, et al: The Team Handbook. Madison, Wis, Joiner Associates, 1988.

33. Lotke E: The prison-industrial complex, Multinatl Monit 17:18-21, 1996.

34. Palmer RH, Hargraves JL, Orav EJ, et al: Leadership for quality improvement in group practices, Med Care 34:SS40-SS51, 1996.

NCCHC Accreditation

Accreditation by the National Commission on Correctional Health Care is a process of external peer review in which NCCHC, an independent organization dedicated to supporting and improving correctional health care, grants public recognition to detention and correctional institutions that meet its nationally recognized *Standards for Health Services.*

Through accreditation, NCCHC renders a professional judgment on the effectiveness of a correctional facility's health services delivery system and assists in its continued improvement in this area.

NCCHC accreditation confers many benefits. It promotes an efficient and well-managed health care delivery system. It adds to the prestige of the facility, increases staff morale, aids recruiting efforts, helps to obtain community support, and provides additional justification for budgetary requests. Accreditation also can help protect a facility's assets by minimizing the occurrence of adverse events. In many instances, accreditation can help reduce liability premiums and protect facilities from lawsuits related to health care.

In addition, accreditation benefits the health of the public, staff, and juveniles by assuring that those incarcerated receive adequate and appropriate health care as recommended by the leading authorities in the country.

The Application Process

Call, write, or visit our website to obtain an accreditation application. NCCHC accredits individual correctional facilities; thus, the application must be signed by the person legally responsible for the facility. Upon receipt, we will send you a self-survey questionnaire (SSQ). Information provided on the SSQ is reviewed by NCCHC staff and is used to help you prepare for the on-site survey. NCCHC staff are always available to assist you in its preparation.

Scheduling the Survey

The survey will be scheduled only when you feel you are ready and generally not before 3 to 6 months after your completed SSQ is submitted. Before coming on site we will inform you of the anticipated duration of the survey, which varies based on your facility's size and organization. The average survey lasts two to three days. You also will receive the names of the surveyors well ahead of the site visit. Please make the arrangements necessary for them to enter the facility. If you require additional information for their clearance, simply let us know ahead of time.

The Survey

The accreditation survey should be viewed as a professional learning experience for your staff. NCCHC's survey teams are composed of highly experienced correctional health professionals and always include at least one physician. Our surveyor training is the most rigorous in our field. We verify the credentials, experience, and qualifications of each surveyor, and then provide initial and annual training to ensure that they possess the knowledge and preparation needed to apply the standards to your facility.

Surveyors will try to minimize disruption to your regular activities. In addition to a tour of the facility and entrance and exit conferences with key personnel, the survey includes an extensive review of medical records and other documents, including your policies and procedures. It also includes structured interviews with health staff, administrators, custody staff, and juveniles.

During the entrance conference, the survey team meets with key personnel to discuss the logistics and plan for the survey. Appointments are made and schedules are confirmed for tours, interviews, and the exit conference. The exit conference is intended to provide preliminary feedback about the survey and to answer your questions. Accreditation decisions are not rendered during the exit conference.

After the survey, the survey team submits a report to NCCHC's accreditation committee. The committee will evaluate compliance with the standards and make an accreditation decision. You will receive a comprehensive written report that includes recommendations to assist your compliance with the standards. The accreditation process is designed to be educational for you and your staff, and we will work with you to help you achieve compliance with the standards.

Compliance With Standards

Each of NCCHC's standards is classified as either "essential" or "important." Accredited juvenile detention and confinement facilities are expected to be in compliance with all of the applicable essential standards and at least 85% of the applicable important standards. Generally, essential standards are more directly related to the health, safety, and welfare of patients and the critical components of a health care system (e.g., receiving screening, health assessment, quality assurance). Important standards represent recognized, acceptable practices for health care providers. Whether classified as essential or important, some standards may not apply in a particular situation. For example, facilities that house only male juveniles would not have to demonstrate compliance with Y-G-07 Care of the Pregnant Juvenile.

Accreditation Decisions

The data and other information collected as part of the survey are carefully reviewed by NCCHC's accreditation committee. Depending on the type of application, the decision will be one of the following:

Survey Finding	Initial Application	Continuing Application
Significant compliance	Accreditation	Accreditation
Minimal noncompliance	Accreditation upon verification (AV)	Accreditation upon verification (CAV)
Significant noncompliance	Deferral	Probation
Consistent noncompliance	Denial	Withdrawal

The accreditation committee meets three times a year, usually at the end of February, June, and October. Within approximately 2 weeks of the meeting, NCCHC will send a letter with the accreditation decision and the survey report to the legally responsible person and the health services administrator.

The committee accredits juvenile facilities that demonstrate consistent and significant compliance to the standards. This accomplishment is highly regarded in the fields of health and corrections and those that achieve it are justifiably proud. Facilities that are awarded accreditation will be sent a handsomely framed certificate for display.

Survey Cycle

The usual survey cycle is at least every 3 years. The Accreditation Committee may schedule focused surveys or resurveys more frequently, at its discretion. All facilities, including those scheduled for survey, are required to return an Annual Maintenance Report to confirm continuing compliance with the *Standards* and to provide updates on relevant information.

Accreditation Fees

Accreditation fees are based on sliding scales that factor in the type of facility, average daily population, presence of satellites and their distance from the main facility, and complexity of programs offered. There is an initial accreditation fee and annual fees thereafter. Invoices are sent early in each calendar year.

Additional Information

For the most current information and for additional background and details on the accreditation process, please visit www.ncchc.org, email us at accreditation@ncchc.org, or call 773-880-1460.

Certified Correctional Health Professional Program

Becoming a Certified Correctional Health Professional (CCHP) is the next step in your professional advancement. It is a step toward increased knowledge, greater professional recognition, and identification as a leader in the complex and ever-changing field of correctional health care.

The rewards of a career in correctional health care are many: experience with a wide variety of patients, playing an important role in public health, and working with other dedicated professionals, to name just a few. But health professionals working in correctional settings also face unique challenges: working within strict security regulations, dealing with crowded facilities, understanding the complex legal and public health considerations of providing care to incarcerated populations, and more. Achieving professional certification is the surest way to prove to yourself and to others that you have the tools to meet these challenges.

The CCHP designation identifies you as one who has demonstrated mastery of national standards and the knowledge expected of leaders working in the field of correctional health care. Apply today and join the thousands of correctional health care professionals who have earned the distinction of CCHP.

Benefits of CCHP Certification

CCHP professional certification provides immeasurable benefits and is highly regarded by management, peers, staff, and others. CCHPs use their credential on letterhead, business cards, and all forms of address. In some employment settings, CCHP certification is rewarded financially. Additionally, CCHPs receive the following:

- Certificate suitable for framing
- Lapel or tie pin with the CCHP insignia
- Press release to send to employee newsletters and local media
- Special networking and publishing opportunities
- Discounted membership in the Academy of Correctional Health Professionals

Eligibility Requirements

Professionals from many different disciplines and work settings have earned the CCHP designation. All correctional health professionals who meet the following eligibility requirements are encouraged to apply.

- Credentials appropriate to the applicant's field and employment position, and the requirements of the state in which the applicant is licensed. The credentials must be free of any restriction that would limit professional practice solely to the correctional setting. If a license or credential is not required for practice, then the credential is not required for certification.
- Good character and fitness. Character and fitness is one of the most important components of the application. An applicant's record of conduct should justify the trust of patients, employers, and others.
- Successful completion of the CCHP examination

From time to time, eligibility requirements may be modified or adopted by the CCHP Board of Trustees at its sole discretion. The most current and complete definitions of the eligibility requirements are available on our website at www.ncchc.org/cchp.

Elements of the Application

*   Application form
*   Resume or curriculum vitae documenting education and professional experience
*   Copies of valid credentials, e.g., license, diploma (see eligibility requirements)
*   Signed application statement
*   Appropriate examination fees
*   Exam registration form (provided by NCCHC upon receipt of the above)

Candidacy

When all elements have been received and the application has been approved, applicants will receive acknowledgment of their candidacy to take the CCHP examination. Incomplete applications will be kept on file for six months, after which time persons seeking certification will need to submit a new application and fees. A candidate must take the exam within one year of the application approval date or the closest date to one year that the next exam is administered.

The Examination

Persons who meet the basic eligibility and application requirements participate in a proctored, written examination composed of 80 to 100 multiple-choice questions. Candidates are allowed two hours to complete the examination.

The purpose of the CCHP examination is to measure a candidate's knowledge, understanding, and application of standards and guidelines essential to the delivery of appropriate health care, the basic legal principles for practicing within a correctional health care system, the ethical obligations of correctional health care professionals, and the role of health care professionals in delivering health care in the correctional environment. The examination is not intended to measure clinical competency. Some questions are geared toward specific correctional settings (e.g., jail, prison, or juvenile facility); others are more general in nature.

Candidates will receive their examination results in writing. Candidates who fail to receive a passing score may take the exam two additional times within a two-year period from the date of the initial application approval. The reexamination fee is $45.

Preparing to Take the Examination

The CCHP Board of Trustees has developed a handbook that is sent to all applicants to help them prepare for the examination. You also may download the Candidate Handbook at www.ncchc.org/cchp.

The handbook provides a detailed list of content areas covered on the examination. It does not contain the study materials but instead is a resource to help direct your studies. Test your knowledge by answer sample questions provided at the CCHP website.

The following publications contain the material covered on the examination. We strongly recommend that you study these books to improve examination performance.
*   *Standards for Health Services in Prisons*
*   *Standards for Health Services in Jails*
*   *Standards for Health Services in Juvenile Detention and Confinement Facilities*
*   *Correctional Health Care: Guidelines for the Management of an Adequate Delivery System*

These books may be purchased from NCCHC as a discounted CCHP Study Package or individually. Although the difference between prison and jail health care delivery is significant, there is much overlap in the jail and prison standards, so you might consider purchasing only one of the two. See the NCCHC catalog (www.ncchc.org/pubs) or call 773-880-1460 to order. Alternatively, your employer, colleagues, or library may have these resources. Many CCHP candidates study together and share one set of materials.

Examination Dates and Locations

Examinations are offered several times a year, including at NCCHC conferences. Regional exams are offered at locations where there is a qualified CCHP candidate and a qualified proctor; we will try to make reasonable accommodations for candidates who are farther than a three-hour drive from a test center. Information on how to request a regional test center is enclosed in the confirmation packet; requests must be made at least 90 days before the exam date. The most up-to-date schedule and locations are available at www.ncchc.org/cchp.

ADA Compliance

The CCHP program makes every effort to ensure that test centers are in compliance with the Americans with Disabilities Act. Candidates who require special accommodations must submit a written request at least 90 days before the examination date.

Continuing Certification

Persons who receive a passing score on the examination are awarded certification, which is valid for one year. CCHPs must apply for continuing certification with the Board of Trustees annually. Continuing certification requires participation in 18 hours of continuing education (at least six of which are specific to correctional health care) and payment of the $75 recertification fee. Reexamination is not required. A new certificate that indicates continued certification will be sent.

Advanced Certification (CCHP-A)

Certified Correctional Health Professionals are eligible to apply for advanced certification after three years in the certification program. The advanced program recognizes CCHPs who have demonstrated excellence, commitment, and contribution to the field of correctional health care and their relative discipline or profession. Advanced certification requires the completion of a more detailed application and a passing score on a four-hour, proctored essay examination. Applications are accepted on an ongoing basis. The examination is administered three times a year at the three national NCCHC conferences.

Registered Nurse Certification (CCHP-RN)

Certified Correctional Health Professionals are eligible to apply for registered nurse certification at any time, as long as certification is current. The registered nurse program recognizes CCHPs who have demonstrated the ability to deliver specialized nursing care in corrections. CCHP-RN certification requires the completion of a detailed application and a passing score on a two-hour, proctored, multiple-choice examination. Applications are accepted on an ongoing basis. The examination is administered throughout the year. For the most up-to-date information, please visit www.ncchc.org/cchprn.

Governance of the CCHP Program

The Certified Correctional Health Professional program is governed by a Board of Trustees comprised of 10 correctional health care experts from a variety of health professions. Three of the trustees are elected by their peers; the others are appointed from the correctional health care field. The CCHP Board of Trustees is responsible for examination content, scoring, and evaluation, as well as awarding certification to successful candidates. The CCHP program is administered by the National Commission on Correctional Health Care.

Additional Information

For additional or the most current information on certification, please visit www.ncchc.org/cchp, email us at cchp@ncchc.org, or call 773-880-1460.

GLOSSARY

ACCESS TO CARE means that in a timely manner, a patient can be seen by a clinician, be given a professional clinical judgment, and receive care that is ordered.

ACTIVITIES OF DAILY LIVING (ADL) generally refers to ambulation, bathing, dressing, feeding, and toileting.

ADMINISTRATIVE REVIEW is an assessment of correctional and emergency response actions surrounding a juvenile's death. Its purpose is to identify areas where facility operations, policies, and procedures can be improved.

ADOLESCENCE is defined as the period of life that begins with puberty and ends with completed growth and physical maturity, and requires special attention to exercise, nutrition, and appropriate social interaction.

ADVANCE DIRECTIVES are expressions of the patient's wishes as to how future care should be delivered or declined, including decisions that must be made when the patient is not capable of expressing those wishes. Examples include living wills, which specify what the patient wants done; health care proxies, which specify who can make decisions for the patient when the patient is incapacitated; and a DNR order, which is a patient's specific refusal of certain extraordinary measures that may prolong life. It should be noted that these terms may differ from state to state depending on the language used in legislation and court decisions.

ADVERSE CLINICAL EVENT is defined as an injury or death caused by medical management rather than by the patient's underlying disease or condition. A sizable proportion of adverse events in the community are the result of human errors. For example, switching two look-alike medications (e.g., Prozac and Doxipen) is a potentially easy mistake. Giving the wrong medication to patients during pill line administration is an adverse clinical event.

AIDS TO IMPAIRMENT are devices such as eyeglasses, hearing aids, canes, crutches, and wheelchairs that enhance or restore physical functions.

AUTOMATED EXTERNAL DEFIBRILLATORS (AEDs) are electronic devices that interpret cardiac rhythms and, if necessary, deliver an electrical shock to the patient.

CHEMICAL DEPENDENCY refers to the state of physiological and/or psychological dependence on alcohol, opium derivatives, synthetic drugs with morphine-like properties (opiates), stimulants, and depressants.

CHILD CARE STAFF includes line security as well as correctional administration.

CHRONIC DISEASE is an illness or condition that affects an individual's well-being for an extended interval, usually at least 6 months, and generally is not curable but can be managed to provide optimum functioning within any limitations the condition imposes on the individual.

CHRONIC DISEASE PROGRAM incorporates a treatment plan and regular clinic visits. The clinician monitors the patient's progress during clinic visits and, when necessary, changes the treatment. The program also includes patient education for symptom management.

CLINICAL ENCOUNTERS are interactions between patients and health care professionals that involve a treatment and/or an exchange of confidential information.

CLINICAL MORTALITY REVIEW is an assessment of the clinical care provided and the circumstances leading up to a death. Its purpose is to identify areas of patient care or system policies and procedures that can be improved.

CLINICAL PERFORMANCE ENHANCEMENT is the process of having a health professional's work reviewed by another professional of at least equal training in the same general discipline, such as the review of the facility's physicians by the responsible physician.

CLINICAL PRACTICE GUIDELINES, according to the National Academy of Sciences' Institute of Medicine, are systematically developed, science-based statements designed to assist clinician and patient with decisions about appropriate health care for specific clinical circumstances. Clinical practice guidelines are used to assist clinical decision making, assess and assure the quality of care, provide education about clinical disease, guide the allocation of health care resources, and reduce the risk of legal liability for negligent care.

NATIONAL CLINICAL PRACTICE GUIDELINES are those presented by national professional organizations and accepted by experts in the respective medical field. (NCCHC's clinical guidelines are available at www.ncchc.org.)

CLINICAL SETTING refers to an examination or treatment room appropriately supplied and equipped to address the patient's health care needs.

CLINICALLY ORDERED RESTRAINT is a therapeutic intervention initiated by medical or mental health staff to use devices designed to safely limit a patient's mobility.

CLINICALLY ORDERED SECLUSION is a therapeutic intervention initiated by medical or mental health staff to use rooms designed to safely limit a patient's mobility.

CLINICIAN'S CLINIC is sick call held by physicians, nurse practitioners, physician assistants, dentists, or mental health clinicians.

COMMUNICABLE DISEASES include those transmitted sexually, through the respiratory system, or by infected blood (e.g., syphilis, gonorrhea, chlamydia, HIV, tuberculosis, hepatitis).

COMPREHENSIVE HEALTH SUMMARIES are documents containing relevant health information including medical, dental, and mental health diagnoses, medications, significant chronic conditions, and pending health referrals.

CONTINUOUS QUALITY IMPROVEMENT (CQI)

BASIC CQI PROGRAM includes monitoring the fundamental aspects of the facility's health care system through one outcome study and one process study (e.g., access to care, the intake process, continuity of care, emergency care and hospitalizations, adverse patient occurrences including all deaths) at least annually.

COMPREHENSIVE CQI PROGRAM includes a multidisciplinary quality improvement committee, monitoring of the areas specified in the compliance indicators, and an annual review of the effectiveness of the CQI program itself. In addition, the program includes two process quality improvement studies and two outcome quality improvement studies, and both studies identify areas in need of improvement and effect remedial actions or strategies.

MULTIDISCIPLINARY QUALITY IMPROVEMENT COMMITTEE is a group of health staff from various disciplines (e.g., medicine, nursing, mental health, dentistry, health records, pharmacy, laboratory) that designs quality improvement monitoring activities, discusses the results, and implements corrective action.

OUTCOME QUALITY IMPROVEMENT STUDIES examine whether expected outcomes of patient care were achieved.

PROCESS QUALITY IMPROVEMENT STUDIES examine the effectiveness of the health care delivery process.

CRITIQUES of drills or actual events document activities including response time, names and titles of health staff, and the roles and responses of all participants. The critique contains observations of appropriate and inappropriate staff response to the drill.

DAILY means 7 days a week including holidays.

DEGREE OF DISEASE CONTROL refers to how well the disease or illness is being treated so that the symptoms do not interfere with daily living and related complications do not develop.

DENTAL. See Oral.

DESIGNATED MENTAL HEALTH CLINICIAN refers to a psychiatrist, psychologist, or psychiatric social worker who is responsible for clinical mental health issues when mental health services at the facility are under a different authority than the medical services.

DETOXIFICATION is the process by which an individual is gradually withdrawn from a drug by the administration of decreasing doses of the drug on which the person is physiologically dependent, of one that is cross-tolerant to it, or of one that medical research has demonstrated to be effective.

DEVELOPMENTALLY DISABLED INDIVIDUALS include those with limited intellectual ability who may need habilitation planning, assistance in accepting the limitations of their conditions, and special attention to their physical safety in the corrections environment.

DIAGNOSTIC SERVICES include biomedical or imaging services and results that are used to make clinical judgments. These diagnostic services may be provided by reference laboratories, hospital radiology and laboratory departments, public health agencies, or correctional facilities.

DIALYSIS PATIENTS are those with end-stage renal disease requiring hemodialysis or peritoneal dialysis on a recurrent basis.

DISCHARGE PLANNING refers to the process of providing sufficient medications and arranging for necessary follow-up health services before the inmate's release to the community.

DRUG ENFORCEMENT AGENCY (DEA)-CONTROLLED SUBSTANCES are the medications that come under the jurisdiction of the Federal Controlled Substances Act.

EARLY RELEASE refers to the release of a juvenile before the expiration of his or her sentence based on the juvenile's terminal condition. In some states, this is known as medical parole or compassionate release.

ECTOPARASITES such as pediculosis and scabies are parasites that live on the skin. They are communicable and may lead to secondary infections.

EMERGENCY HEALTH CARE (medical, mental health, and dental) is care for an acute illness or an unexpected health need that cannot be deferred until the next scheduled sick call or clinic.

EMERGENCY RESPONSE PLAN is the plan developed to respond to manmade or natural, internal or external disasters. It includes, at least, health aspects of an emergency plan, among other items, include the triaging process, outlining where care can be provided, and laying out a backup plan.

ERROR REPORTING SYSTEM includes policies and procedures that outline how health staff voluntarily identify and report all clinical errors, whether the error occurs by omission (failing to do something that is supposed to be done) or commission (doing something that is not supposed to be done).

EXERCISE is increased aerobic activity that stimulates and improves physical and mental health through the use of large-muscle activities such as walking, jogging in place, basketball, and isometrics.

EXPOSURE CONTROL PLAN describes staff actions to be taken to eliminate or minimize exposures to pathogens.

FORENSIC INFORMATION is physical or psychological data collected from an inmate that may be used against him or her in disciplinary or legal proceedings.

FORMULARY is a written list of prescription and nonprescription medications that are ordinarily available to authorized prescribers, including consultants, working for the facility.

FRAGILE JUVENILES include those who suffer from conditions that impair their ability to function to the extent that they require assistance in activities of daily living (e.g., dressing, feeding, transferring, toileting).

HEALTH ADMINISTRATOR is a person who by virtue of education, experience, or certification (e.g., MSN, MPH, MHA, FACHE, CCHP) is capable of assuming responsibility for arranging all levels of health care and ensuring quality and accessible health services for inmates.

HEALTH ASSESSMENT is the process whereby an individual's health status is evaluated, including questioning the patient about symptoms. The extent of the health assessment is defined by the responsible physician but should include at least the steps noted in standard Y-E-04.

HEALTH CARE is the sum of all actions, preventive and therapeutic, taken for the physical and mental well-being of a population. Health care includes medical, dental, mental health, nutrition, and other ancillary services, as well as maintaining clean and safe environmental conditions.

HEALTH CARE LIAISON generally carries out the following duties: reviewing receiving screening forms for follow-up attention; triaging nonemergency sick-call requests every 24 hours; facilitating sick call by having juveniles and records available for the health care professional; and helping to carry out clinicians' orders regarding such matters as diet, housing, and work assignments. The health care liaison may be a child care worker or other person without a health care license who is trained by the responsible physician in limited aspects of health care coordination.

HEALTH CHECKS are face-to-face encounters with the segregated juvenile to ascertain medical and mental health status and provide an opportunity for requests for health care. When problems are noted, appropriate clinical interventions are initiated that may include the discontinuation of segregation for health reasons.

HEALTH EDUCATION is information on preventing illness and maintaining a healthy lifestyle.

HEALTH STAFF includes all qualified health care professionals as well as administrative and support staff (e.g., health record administrators, laboratory technicians, nursing and medical assistants, clerical workers).

HEART-HEALTHY DIET refers to foods that are low in saturated fat, cholesterol, and sodium and high in fiber as promoted by the American Heart Association.

HOSPICE PROGRAM delivers palliative care (medical care and support services aimed at providing comfort). Treatment is focused on symptom control and quality of life issues rather than attempting to cure conditions.

INDEPENDENT REVIEW is the assessment of a health care professional's compliance with discipline-specific and community standards. The review includes an analysis of trends in a practitioner's clinical practice. This review may be conducted by someone who may or may not be directly employed by the facility, as long as the reviewing practitioner has not been previously involved in the care of the patient(s) involved.

INFECTION CONTROL practices are defined by the American Dental Association and the Centers for Disease Control and Prevention as including sterilizing instruments, disinfecting equipment, and properly disposing of hazardous waste.

INFIRMARY is an area in the facility accommodating patients for a period of 24 hours or more, expressly set up and operated for the purpose of caring for patients who need skilled nursing care but do not need hospitalization or placement in a licensed nursing facility, and whose care cannot be managed safely in an outpatient setting. It is not the area itself but the scope of care provided that makes the bed an infirmary bed.

INFIRMARY CARE is care provided to patients with an illness or diagnosis that requires daily monitoring, medication and/or therapy, or assistance with activities of daily living at a level needing skilled nursing intervention..

INFORMED CONSENT is the agreement by a patient to a treatment, examination, or procedure after the patient receives the material facts about the nature, consequences, and risks of the proposed treatment, examination, or procedure; the alternatives to it; and the prognosis if the proposed action is not undertaken.

INTAKE SCREENING. See Receiving Screening.

INTELLECTUAL FUNCTIONING SCREENING includes inquiry into history of developmental and educational difficulties and, when indicated, referral for application of standardized psychological intelligence tools as appropriate.

INTRASYSTEM TRANSFERS include juveniles being transferred from one facility to another within the same correctional authority's system.

ISOLATION. See Segregation.

JUVENILE-DOWN DRILL is a simulated emergency affecting one individual who needs immediate medical intervention. It involves life-threatening situations commonly experienced in correctional settings.

MASS DISASTER DRILL is a simulated emergency involving multiple casualties that require triage by health staff. It frequently involves a natural disaster (e.g., tornado, flood, earthquake), an internal disaster (e.g., riot, arson, kitchen explosion), or external disaster (e.g., mass arrests, bomb threat, power outage).

MEDICAL CLEARANCE is a clinical assessment of physical and mental status before an individual is admitted into the facility. Correctional officers quickly inspect individuals to determine who may be too ill to wait for routine screening or be admitted. Those identified to get immediate medical clearance are pulled from the group prior to admission. The medical clearance may come from on-site health staff or may require sending the individual to the local hospital emergency room. The medical clearance is to be documented in writing.

MEDICAL DIETS are special diets ordered for temporary or permanent health conditions that restrict the types, preparation, and/or amounts of food. Examples include restricted calorie, low sodium, low fat, pureed, soft, liquid, and nutritional supplementation diets.

MEDICAL ISOLATION means housing in a separate room with a separate toilet, hand-washing facility, soap, and single-service towels, and with appropriate accommodations for showering.

MEDICAL RESTRAINT. See Clinically Ordered Restraint.

MEDICATION:

ACCOUNTING is the act of recording, summarizing, analyzing, verifying, and reporting medication usage.

ADMINISTERING medication is the act in which a single dose of an identified drug is given to a patient.

DISPENSING is the placing of one or more doses of a prescribed medication into containers that are correctly labeled to indicate the name of the patient, the contents of the container, and all other vital information.

DISPOSAL is (a) the destruction of medication on its expiration date or when retention is no longer necessary or suitable (e.g., upon patient discharge from the facility), or (b) the provision of medication to the juvenile upon discharge from the facility (in accordance with the continuity-of-care principle).

DISTRIBUTION is the system for delivering, storing, and accounting for medications from the source of supply to the nursing station or point where they are administered to the patient.

ERRORS include errors of commission (wrong medication to patient, wrong dose of medication to patient, wrong schedule for medication, and wrong method of administration) and omission (prescribed medication not given).

FORCED MEDICATIONS are those given without the patient's consent.

PROCURING is the act of ordering medications for the facility.

MENTAL HEALTH SERVICES include the use of a variety of psychosocial and pharmacological therapies, either individual or group, including biological, psychological, and social, to alleviate symptoms, attain appropriate functioning, and prevent relapse.

MENTAL HEALTH STAFF include qualified health care professionals who have received instruction and supervision in identifying and interacting with individuals in need of mental health services.

MORTALITY REVIEW. See Clinical Mortality Review and Administrative Review.

NEAR-MISS CLINICAL EVENT is an error in clinical activity without a consequential adverse patient outcome. For example, a wrong drug is dispensed but not administered to a patient.

NURSING ASSESSMENT PROTOCOLS are written instructions or guidelines that specify the steps to be taken in evaluating a patient's health status and providing interventions. Such protocols may include acceptable first-aid procedures for the identification and care of ailments that ordinarily would be treated by an individual with over-the-counter medication or through self-care. They also may address more serious symptoms such as chest pain, shortness of breath, or intoxication. They specify a sequence of steps to be taken to evaluate and stabilize the patient until a clinician is contacted and orders are received for further care.

OBSERVATION BEDS are beds designated for medical or mental observation for specific purposes, such as watching the patient's response to a change in medication regimen. Patients also can be placed in observation beds to prevent them from eating or drinking before a medical test that requires such restriction, to allow patients to recover from day surgeries or medical procedures, or to watch the general behavior of juveniles whose mental stability appears questionable.

OPIATES are any preparation or derivative of opium, as well as opioid, a synthetic narcotic that resembles an opiate in action but is not derived from opium.

ORAL CARE includes instruction in oral hygiene, examination, and treatment of dental problems. Instruction in oral hygiene minimally includes information on plaque control and the proper brushing of teeth.

ORAL EXAMINATION by a dentist includes taking or reviewing the patient's oral history, an extraoral head and neck examination, charting of teeth, and examination of the hard and soft tissue of the oral cavity with a mouth mirror, explorer, and adequate illumination.

ORAL HYGIENE includes measures to assist the patient in caring for his or her own oral health, including information on plaque control, and the proper brushing and flossing of teeth.

ORAL SCREENING includes visual observation of the teeth and gums, and notation of any obvious or gross abnormalities requiring immediate referral to a dentist.

ORAL TREATMENT includes the full range of services that in the supervising dentist's judgment are necessary for proper mastication and maintaining the juvenile's health status.

ORIENTATION

BASIC ORIENTATION, which is provided on the first day of employment, includes information necessary for the health staff member (e.g., full-time, part-time, consultant, per diem) to function safely in the institution.

IN-DEPTH ORIENTATION includes a full familiarization with the health services delivery system at the facility, and focuses on the similarities and differences between providing health care in the community and in a correctional setting.

ORTHOSES are specialized mechanical devices, such as braces, foot inserts, and hand splints, used to support or supplement weakened or abnormal joints or limbs.

PATIENT SAFETY SYSTEMS are practice interventions designed to prevent adverse or near-miss clinical events. For example, during administration of medications, use of a photo identification system helps to ensure that the right person receives the right drug.

PEER REVIEW. See Clinical Performance Enhancement.

PHYSICAL DISABILITIES can refer to mobility impairments (e.g., amputations, paraplegia) or to other disabilities that limit daily functioning (e.g., visual, hearing, or speech impairments).

PHYSICAL EXAMINATION is an objective, hands-on evaluation of an individual. It involves the inspection, palpation, auscultation, and percussion of a patient's body to determine the presence or absence of physical signs of disease.

PHYSICIAN CLINICAL CHART REVIEW is an evaluation by a physician of the timeliness and appropriateness of the clinical care provided to patients. The number and frequency of chart reviews are expected to increase if significant problems are identified.

POLICY is a facility's official position on a particular issue related to an organization's operations.

POSITION is a job filled by a specific staff member (e.g., medical records secretary, physician, chief nurse). A position has tasks that can usually be deferred until the staff member is available.

POST is a job defined by its location, time, and duties that can be filled interchangeably by different staff members (e.g., 7-3 infirmary nurse). Continuous coverage usually distinguishes a post from a position; a post has tasks that cannot usually be deferred.

POTENTIALLY SUICIDAL inmates are not actively suicidal but express suicidal ideation and/or have a recent history of self-destructive behavior.

PRESCRIBING CLINICIAN is a licensed individual, such as an MD, DO, NP, or PA, authorized to write prescriptions.

PRIMARY CARE, according to the National Academy of Sciences' Institute of Medicine, is the provision of integrated, accessible health care services by clinicians who are accountable for addressing a large majority of personal health care needs, developing a sustained partnership with patients, and practicing in the context of family and community.

PRIMARY CARE CLINICIANS are all licensed practitioners providing the facility's primary care; this includes medical physicians, psychiatrists, dentists, midlevel practitioners (i.e., nurse practitioners, physician assistants), and PhD-level psychologists.

PROCEDURE describes in detail, sometimes in sequence, how a policy is to be carried out.

PROSTHESES are artificial devices to replace missing body parts such as limbs, teeth, eyes, or heart valves.

PSYCHOLOGICAL AUTOPSY, sometimes referred to as a PSYCHOLOGICAL RECONSTRUCTION and usually conducted by a psychologist or other qualified mental health professional, is a written reconstruction of an individual's life with an emphasis on factors that may have contributed to the death.

QUALIFIED HEALTH CARE PROFESSIONALS include physicians, physician assistants, nurses, nurse practitioners, dentists, mental health professionals, and others who by virtue of their education, credentials, and experience are permitted by law to evaluate and care for patients.

QUALIFIED MENTAL HEALTH PROFESSIONALS include psychiatrists, psychologists, psychiatric social workers, psychiatric nurses, and others who by virtue of their education, credentials, and experience are permitted by law to evaluate and care for the mental health needs of patients.

QUALITY IMPROVEMENT. See Continuous Quality Improvement.

RECEIVING SCREENING is a process of structured inquiry and observation of all inmates being admitted, designed to obtain immediate treatment for inmates who are in need of emergency health care, identify and meet ongoing current health needs, and isolate those with communicable diseases.

REQUEST for health care refers to oral or written petitions for medical, dental, or mental health services.

RESPONSIBLE HEALTH AUTHORITY (RHA) is responsible for the facility's health care services, and arranges for all levels of health care and assures quality, accessible, and timely health services for inmates. The RHA may be a physician, *health administrator*, or agency.

RESPONSIBLE PHYSICIAN is a designated MD or DO who has the final authority at a given facility regarding clinical issues.

RESTRAINT. See Clinically Ordered Restraint.

RESTRICTED LICENSES refers to licenses that have attached stipulations that must be followed. Different state licensing boards refer to these modified licenses by various names including temporary, probation, stipulated order or agreement, practice restriction, institutional, restricted, disciplinary, provisional, limited, and conditional.

SEGREGATED JUVENILES are those isolated from the general population and who receive services and activities apart from other juveniles. Facilities may refer to juveniles housed in such conditions as being in administrative segregation, protective custody, or disciplinary segregation.

SELF-CARE is care for a condition that can be treated by the juvenile and may include over-the-counter medications.

SELF-MEDICATION PROGRAMS (also known as keep-on-person programs) permit responsible juveniles to carry and administer their own medications.

SERIOUS MENTAL HEALTH NEEDS PATIENTS include those with basic psychotic disorders or mood disorders (e.g., manic-depressives), self-mutilators, the aggressive mentally ill, those with posttraumatic stress disorders, and suicidal juveniles.

SEXUAL ASSAULT is a sexual act that is coercive or assaultive in nature and that involves the use or the threat of force.

SHELTERED HOUSING, as opposed to infirmary or observation beds, provides a protective environment that does not require 24-hour nursing care. The beds can be in the infirmary itself or in other designated areas (e.g., where hospice-level care or "step-down" or transitional mental health care is provided). Sheltered housing is equivalent to home care for those not confined to an institutional setting.

SICK CALL is the evaluation and treatment of an ambulatory patient in a clinical setting, either on or off site, by a qualified health care professional.

SPECIAL NEEDS PATIENTS include those with chronic diseases or conditions that require regular care.

SPECIALTY CARE means specialist-provided health care (e.g., nephrology, surgery, dermatology, orthopedics).

STAFF SAFETY refers to the health and well-being of health staff who work in the facility. It is directly related to the administrative practice that assures public safety of the facility.

STAFFING PLAN lays out the full-time equivalent (FTE) staff coverage required, lists current incumbents and vacancies, and addresses how full coverage will be accomplished if all positions are not filled (e.g., use of agency, temporary, or part-time staff). A staffing plan is a detailed schedule on which classifications of staff are assigned to posts and positions for the health care unit.

STANDARD PRECAUTIONS combine the major features of universal precautions (designed to reduce the risk of transmission of bloodborne pathogens) and body secretion isolation (designed to reduce the transmission of pathogens from moist body substances) and apply them to all patients receiving care, regardless of their diagnosis or presumed infection status.

STANDING ORDERS are written orders that specify the same course of treatment for each patient suspected of having a given condition, and that specify the use and amount of prescription drugs.

SUICIDAL. See Potentially Suicidal.

TABLETOP EXERCISES are discussions about health staff's projected response to emergencies.

TERMINALLY ILL JUVENILE is one whose physical condition has deteriorated to the point where the prognosis is less than a year to live.

TRAINING. See Orientation.

TREATMENT PLAN is a series of written statements specifying a patient's particular course of therapy and the roles of qualified health care professionals in carrying it out.

TRIAGE is the sorting and classifying of juveniles' health requests to determine priority of need and the proper place for health care to be rendered.

UNIVERSAL PRECAUTIONS. See Standard Precautions.

VIOLENT BEHAVIOR is defined as EXPRESSIVE VIOLENCE initiated as a result of an interpersonal altercation where the goal is to injure the other person, or as INSTRUMENTAL VIOLENCE where the goal is to get something from the person (usually the result of criminal intent).

WITHIN SIGHT OR HEARING of a qualified health care professional means that the patient can gain the professional's attention through visual or auditory signals. Call lights and buzzer systems can be useful ways to ensure this.

WRITTEN AGREEMENT means a contract, letter of agreement, or memorandum of understanding between the facility and the hospital, clinic, or specialist for the care and treatment of patients.

WRITTEN INFORMATION may take the form of a facility handbook, a handout, or postings in inmate housing areas.

A bold page number indicates the page on which a standard addressing the topic appears.

Immunization 67, 125, 129

Independent review 36, 37, 122

Infection control 7, **23**-25, 43, 45, 46, 72, 73

Infirmary 8, 9, 42, 96, **106**-108, 112, 160

Information on health services **61**

Informed consent and right to refuse 93, 105, 125, 136, **138**-141, 151

See also *Consent*

Initial health assessment 67, 69, 70

Intake screening 64, 111

Intellectual functioning 71

Intoxication and withdrawal 39, 62, 64, 83, 96, **114**-118, 141, 164

See also *Alcohol and other drugs*

See also *Detoxification*

Intrasystem transfers 66, 67

Isolation 23, 24, 46, 64, 78-80, 110

Job description 4

Jurisdictions 15, 145

Juvenile worker 26, **41**, 42

Keep-on-person 49, 50

Kitchen 9, 13, 25-27

Laundry 25, 27, 95

License/licensure 4, 35-38, 43, 44, 55, 57, 72, 73, 84, 92, 167, 168

Licensed nursing facility 107

Lockdown 6, 93, 94

Medical autonomy **5**, 6

Medical clearance 26, 62, 63

Medical isolation 23, 79

See also *Isolation*

Medical parole 121

Medical records See *Health records*

Medical research See *Research*

Medication errors 51-53

Medication services **51**, 85, 136, 160

Medications 23, 28, 29, 39-43, 49-53, 62-64, 70, 72, 76-78, 82-87, 91-93, 96, 101-103, 107, 109, 117, 125, 128, 129, 136, 137, 139, 140, 149, 159, 160

Administration training **40**, 41

Over-the-counter 23, 53, 83, 91

See also *Psychotropics*

Mental health 3, 5, 6, 11, 15, 32, 43, 55, 56, 64, 67, 71, 73, 75-82, 86, 94, 96, 104, 105, 107, 108, 112, 113, 125, 129, 133, 139, 149

Assessment 66, 69, 78

Clinicians 4, 7, 15, 75, 108, 110, 112, 113, 118

Screening and evaluation **70**, 71, 85, 103, 150

Services 4, 7, 8, 18, 53, 54, 71, 75, 80, **109**, 110, 118, 147, 149, 160

Staff 32, 40, 64, 70, 71, 78, 80, 95, 96, 105, 112, 113, 117, 134

See also *Qualified mental health professionals*

Mortality 17, 18, 102

See also *Death*

Near-miss clinical event 28, 29

Nonemergency health care requests and services **74**, 80, 82

Nonformulary 50

Nursing assessment protocols **83**, 84

Nutrition See *Diet*

Observation beds 107

Opioid/opiates 51, 52, 114, 115

Oral health 3, 4, 7, 8, 23, 24, 43, 53, 55, 61, 62, 66, 67, **72**-76, 78, 79, 82, 85, 86, 92, 120, 125, 129, 139, 153, 154, 160, 178

Orientation for health staff 36, **45**, 46, 127, 138

See also *Education of health staff*

Orientation for juveniles See *Education of juveniles*

Orthotic See *Aids to impairment*

Outside programs 39

Peer review 12, 30, 37, 163

See also *Clinical performance enhancement*

Performance measures 65, 66, 69, 77, 81, 106, 113, 114, 135, 157

Perinatal care 92

See also *Prenatal care*

Pharmaceutical operations 40, **49**

Pharmaceuticals See *Medications*

Physical examination 26, 28, 31, 67, 68, 129

Policies and procedures **8**-10

Position, employment 38, 42, 43, 45, 167

Position statement xiii, 3, 36

Post 42, 44, 71

Pregnant 9, 15, 23, 55, 62, 65, 104, 114-117, 119, 150, 164

　　　　A bold page number indicates the page on which a standard addressing the topic appears.